Live Lazy, Live Large

Tips for Making Life Fun for Us Ol' Ladies

A sherrillwark.com WORDPRESS BLOG

Sherrill WARK

Ottawa Canada
crowecreations.ca

A sherrillwark.com WordPress blog © 2021

First Crowe Creations edition August 2021
crowecreations.ca

Designed by Crowe Creations
Text set in Segoe UI; headings set in Backtalk Serif BTN

Cover photo from iStock: Prostock-Studio Stock photo ID:931738852
Cover design © 2021 by Crowe Creations

Illustrations from www.needpix.com
Photos © Sherrill Wark

Crowe Creations
ISBN: 978-1-927058-83-1

To all us old gals.

We ain't dead yet.

The Hypersleep Method

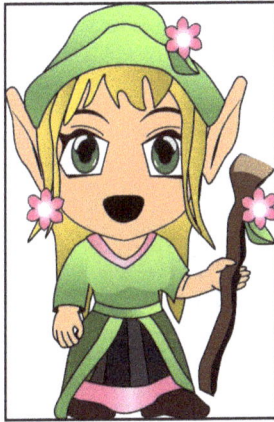

"What is this place? I don't recognize anything."—Ripley, Aliens.

WOULDN'T IT BE MARVELOUS TO WAKE up in the morning and have had the elves in overnight to tidy up the house and to have breakfast on the table already? Well, at least coffee? Oh, and to have done the shopping for you, too?

It's possible. Yes it is. But you won't have to use fairy tale magic. You'll be using a different kind of magic.

Over the next few months, I'll post ideas about how to make your life easier and how to be more organized and thus have oodles of time left over to nap and watch TV.

Let's Go on an Adventure

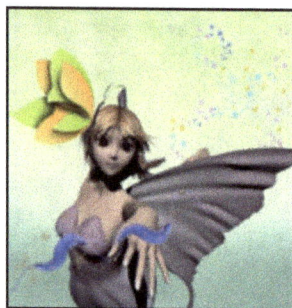

"But to where?"
"Where, indeed?"

PEOPLE OFTEN ASK ME WHERE I get the energy to do everything I do. I don't have any more energy than anyone else. What I have is time. Lots of it.

Where does that time come from?

No. I'm not someone who's all obsessed with routine or schedules. Far from it! I'm a rebel. I don't like to be controlled by anything or anybody. And I think that's why I try to shave time whenever I can. (I just noticed that if you remove a letter from *shave time* you have *save time* or you have *have time*.)

How much time do I have exactly?

24 hours a day

= 8,760 hours a year

= 525,600 minutes a year

= 31,536,000 seconds a year

Same as everybody else on Earth. Imagine that.

I would need to take 10,512,000 seconds a year—give or take—for sleeping. This would leave me with 21,024,000 seconds per year to do whatever I wanted.

How Do I Manage to Keep those 21,024,000 Seconds a Year to Myself?

When I was a kid, we lived in a small town in a really great neighborhood where two dead-end streets crossed. William Street and Peter Street. Both of these streets were dead ends because the gully was there. It curved slightly to be behind both streets.

We moved to that neighborhood when I was six or seven, and out of there when I was about thirteen. I was the eldest of three. My sister was born when I was five-and-a-half and my brother, when I was eleven.

I had thirty-six friends that I played with. I remember that number because one Halloween, to know how many treats she'd have to prepare, Mom counted the kids and came up with thirty-six. I remember the number because I was worrying about what might happen if one of the kids had a cousin staying with them or an extra kid showed up or something. I didn't ask. Mom, I knew, would come up with something.

Those were post-WWII days, the 1950s, so we were all pretty much of the same mentality and even social status. We all got along. Sometimes we didn't get along. But we usually worked it out. We were kids. This was our 'hood.

We played tag. We played scrub (softball); I pretty much ended up as 30th fielder most of the time. We played Hide n Seek. We played Red Rover.

I especially liked playing Cowboys and Indians. I would get especially upset, though, when I couldn't take a turn to play Roy Rogers. One of the boys always got that role. I wasn't upset from missing out because I wanted to be Roy Rogers and couldn't because I was a girl; it was because I wanted to be riding Trigger.

Everybody went to the Saturday Afternoon Matinees. Cowboy movies galore. The kids we knew from school would be there, too. And both Protestants and Catholics from every neighborhood in town. The theater would be full to the brim. Only the older kids got to sit upstairs in the balcony.

In the summer, we would catch bees and grass-hoppers in jars with holes in the lids and in the winter we would risk death—no exaggeration—tobogganing down the gully's hills.

Life was great. Freedom was wonderful. I even liked school. A lot.

Day of Doom

I think I was probably nine when my mother announced that I was now old enough to be doing the dishes on Saturday mornings. And if I wanted to be getting an allowance to go to the movies, I had better agree.

"But Mom. I want to go out and play. It's Saturday morning."

"You can play after you do your chores."

Sigh.

The first thought through my head was an unspoken one: *The neighborhood BOYS don't have to do chores on Saturday morning!* I could hear them all outside playing. I wanted to be there, too. A lot of the neighborhood girls were into dolls. And probably into washing dishes, too. Dolls, to me, were absolutely no fun whatsoever. Doing the dishes even less. I didn't want to play with the girls and do girl stuff. I wanted to do the stuff boys did. That stuff was fun.

The first few times I did the dishes, I had to redo them. Because my hands couldn't tolerate having the water hot enough to make the Tide laundry soap be absorbed and work, I couldn't get the dishes clean enough.

"Do them over, Sherrill. They're still dirty."

You might imagine my reaction to *that*.

I devised a plan.

I need to get the water as hot as I can get it without causing damage to my hands. That way, I won't have to do them over.

If I can get the dishes done faster in the first place, I can get out to play sooner.

How could I do this?

If I set everything up in certain corners in the sink, I would be able to just reach in and grab what I wanted fast. I wouldn't have to deal with the water burning my skin while blindly searching around for a spoon or a fork under sudsy, opaque water. I would know exactly where everything was so I could dive my hand in and come up with whatever needed washing almost instantly. And since I would know where the paring knife was, I could avoid cutting myself. I could even start washing things while the sink was filling up.

It worked!

That was the beginning of my learning how to s/h/ave time. As I said, it wasn't the least bit obsessive-compulsive on my part. It was solely so I could get out and play sooner.

And I'm the same way today: Get it done properly, but *Get 'er done!* and then you can go play.

How Can I Know Exactly Where Everything Is?

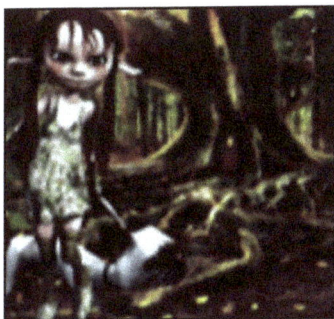

"But..."

HAVE YOU EVER GOTTEN UP IN the middle of the night with this urge for a drink of water or milk or juice or that last chicken wing? Maybe a mouthful of yogurt?

Have you then stumbled through the dark of your apartment or house to the fridge?

How did you know where the fridge was?

You knew because it was exactly where you left it.

Might be a different story though, when you open the fridge door. Do you stand there with the fridge's light gleaming into your eyes to fully waken you from your semi-sleep state so you can hunt around for the orange juice?

What if you had put the orange juice back where it was the last time you used it? What if you always put the orange juice in the same spot in the fridge?

I know exactly where my milk is because I use it in my coffee. Often.

I make a morning's worth of coffee (half a pot?*) because I don't want to waste time waiting for the water in one of those one-at-a-time machines to heat up again; and run through two little pods' worth: one caffeinated and the other not. (I drink my coffee half and half. Decaf isn't worth the water; and if I drink pure caff, it causes my patience to pack up and leave me stranded.)

Plus, I use big coffee mugs so I would need two pods—or maybe one and a half... umm... divided three-quarters and three-quarters... Or maybe three-ish pods? umm... (Who ever said that girls of our time didn't need to learn arithmetic?) Is it going to overflow my mug this time? (Or geometry and physics.) I have to stand there (waste time) and watch...

Sigh.

Nope. As soon the coffee finishes running through, I remove it from the machine and cover it. Covering it is important; there's not much that's worse than stale coffee.

---

*I have recently taken a liking to drinking iced coffee year round so make a whole pot. And this is another reason why one of those one-at-a-time machines don't work for me: I'd have to wait too long for it to cool off, even with milk and ice in it.

Ew. I cover it with a folded dish cloth but I add folded paper towels between it and the pot. Coffee "smoke" stains. (More to wash, more to dry, more to fold = time wasted.)

When I go with non-iced coffee, I heat up my refills in the microwave and while this goes on, I walk around, stretch, look out the window... Because I work. I write books. For my business, Crowe Creations, I edit and design books for Indie authors. I do volunteer work. This means I am sitting at my computer for long stretches of time. I need to get up and walk around and adjust my poor eyeballs and the rest of my body.

It's Not Always Easy But...

I know it's not easy to know exactly where everything is in your home if you have offspring, a spouse, or the equivalent. Even those you hire to clean your house can put something somewhere else. Kitties can flick unattended objects under furniture.

Do you know exactly where your microwave is? Your toaster oven? Why do you know where they are but not your orange juice?

Where are your keys? Could you close your eyes and go put your hand on them right this minute?

Where's your favorite sweater or blankie that you like to use when you're watching TV? Same question: Could you close your eyes and go put your hand on it right this minute?

"One thousand and one. One thousand and two. One thousand and three." Those are wasted seconds if you can't put your hand on your keys or your sweater.

"My keys are in my purse. Where's my stupid purse? Where did I leave it?"

Tick, tick, tick, tick...

We could be watching TV. Reading. Napping. Playing solitaire. Going for a walk/run/bike ride. Shopping (fun-shopping). Lunching or coffee-ing with a friend. Laughing our heads off while sharing jokes on Facebook. Knitting. Crocheting. Sculpting. Drawing. Painting.

I could be writing a book. Gardening. (Even in an apartment, one can garden.) Doing my volunteer work. Writing a blog...

Instead, I'm wandering around in a panic—bringing unhealthy stress into my life—looking for something when I could be having fun.

Someone might say, "C'mon, Sherrill. That's really weird that you always keep everything in the exact same place and always return it to the exact same place. Doesn't that indicate a mental disorder?"

I might respond with, "So... You're saying I should be trying to make sure I put everything in a different place?"

If you want to s/h/ave time, stop wasting time looking for things.

Where Do I Keep Things?

I do my best to keep things in the most logical place for them. The handiest spot. If I use them often, they will be at the forefront of the shelf, drawer or cabinet. As Mr. Spock would say, "It's only logical."

My keys are on top of a small bookcase in the hall near the door. Why would I want to bring them to the living room and put them on the coffee table? Where the cat (when I had a cat) might see them when my back was turned and flick them onto the floor and under the couch?

If you leave something in a place long enough, a cat won't assume it's something new and get the urge to flick it to see what it ends up doing. Curiosity, eh?

And yes. My herbs and spices are in alphabetical order. I have dozens of them so if I don't want to spend ages looking for what goes into the recipe I'm currently working on, I have to set them up that way. This also helps me from purchasing extra packages/bottles of stuff I already had but couldn't find. Like about forty years' worth, now, of rarely used marjoram. Sigh.

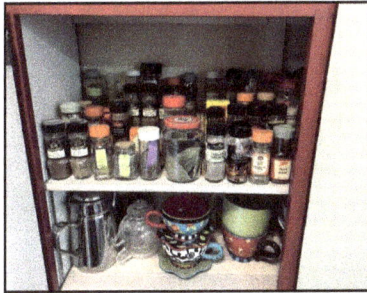

Oops. I see that my little glass teapot with its accompanying glass cup under it is in need of dusting. It's on the shelf below the herbs and spices and between the big silver-colored teapot and the colorful, artistic cups and saucers. See?

(Excuse me... There. Done. Took about 45 seconds to dust that off. So 45 seconds shaved off my spring cleaning when it comes up. Well, maybe 47 seconds if you count opening and closing the cupboard door. [*insert smiley face rolling its eyes*])

Speaking of Cooking and Baking

When I cook or bake anything, I always go through the recipe, get out everything I'll need from my cupboards and have it ready before I start. I measure out the flour ahead of time into a bowl; the herbs/spices go into a small bowl or dish together (if they are called for at the same time in the recipe); the eggs get pre-beaten (at the last moment, eh?); the baking pans are prepared as per instructions...

Then as soon as I use it, back the bottle or package or container or bowl goes to its space.

I clean up as I go. I made bread this morning. Albeit in a bread maker, but still, I had everything lined up.

As I added each ingredient (with a bread maker, one MUST do things in order so the yeast touches neither the sugar nor the water), I washed the utensils/bowls/measuring spoons and popped these things back where they belong.

Then I put the baking pan into its chamber, locked it in, closed the lid, tapped the required button to choose crust color (I had set the time when I plugged it in; why not? I was right there leaning over it anyway), stepped to the sink and washed the little bowl I'd measured the yeast into and the big bowl I'd measured the flour into...

Tada! The elves must have been around. I had nothing more to do, so back to the book I'm writing = having fun. Then on to editing this blog post = having fun.

Where Do I Find Room for "Everything in its Place?"

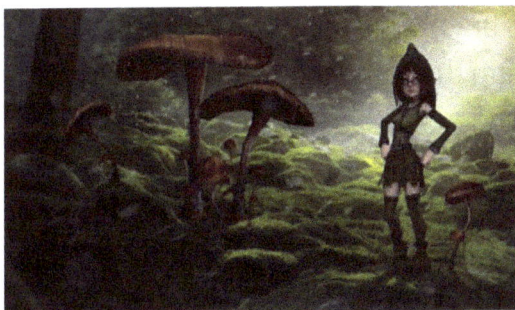

"Every time I turn around, something else has sprouted."

Ah. The age-old question for us older gals who have accumulated too much over the years: Where did it all come from?

And where can I put it?

During Ice Storm '98, I realized there is very little we actually *need*. We *need* oxygen, water, food, and shelter from the elements. Every species on Earth requires these things. (Yes, yes. I know there are "things" that can live in volcanoes, but you know what I mean.)

Do we actually *need* those four big salad bowls that probably still have our name taped on the bottom?

Do we *need* all of those exactly-the-same-size/purpose cooking pots that are now somewhere in the back of that bottom shelf/drawer? Possibly missing a handle or lid? When's the last time we used them all at the same time? Ever?

How many sets of dishes do we *need*?

We are now living alone. No spouse. No kids. Twenty-four hours to ourselves but we never seem to have time to do anything other than what we always did. Here we are, doing the same things over and over as though life hadn't changed in the last ten, twenty, thirty, forty, fifty years...

Times *have* changed. We are old ladies now and we go to *their* place for special occasions. We don't *need* all that extra stuff in our way, using up the time we have left.

It's time to give all those extras to the children.

But perhaps our children are now beginning to downsize. They aren't going to be wanting (needing) all those extra pots and pans and bowls and kitchen gadgets either. They most likely have doubles and triples of their own that they're wanting to rehome.

It's Time

It's time to say farewell to that dear special bowl that holds only memories now instead of potential salad. Memories belong in our hearts, not on the back of a shelf.

If these things are of sentimental value (e.g., something that belonged to Great-Great Granny or Grampy), keep them in the family then. Were we not keeping them to hand down in the first place? It's time.

Instead of keeping everything until we die, thus forcing our grieving children to go through every little thing in our home for days—perhaps even years—let's give them to the kids *now*. Or to the grandchildren.

If we don't have children or grandchildren, we can give them to our brother's or sister's kids/grandkids.

Let's give them the story that goes along with these objects, thus wrapping these treasures in their own preciousness. Let's hand over the responsibility of keeping the memories alive to *them*. Let's tell ourselves it's no longer our responsibility. Let's convince ourselves.

It's time.

It's time to relieve ourselves of the worry and potential guilt that goes along with the assumed responsibility of keeping all the family treasures...

... in the back of the bottom shelf in that cupboard in the kitchen? In a box in the basement? What respect does it get there?

"But I don't have time to sort through everything."

What did you just say? You don't have time?

We are going to dump this chore on our kids when we die?

While they are grieving us?

That's mean.

Even if it won't be our own children, it will be someone's child, whatever age. Someone's child will have to go through every single thing we own and decide what to do with it.

It's time.

It Ain't Easy

When we lose someone, even a kitty, the experience gets filed away in our brains. I like to think of the brain as a big, huge, giant filing cabinet with oodles of drawers. The Grief Drawer is labeled as such.

As you might imagine, words spoken and sights and things seen can trigger memories. Grief's memories. And any time we want to file something in a filing cabinet, we have to open the drawer it will be going into and finger our way through the As and Bs and Cs and Ds...

When we open the Grief Drawer, we see all those labels on all those separate files. "There's Mom. There's Dad. There's my cousin. There's my aunt. There's that guy I liked when I was in Grade 4, killed in a car accident when he was barely nineteen years old. There's my first dog. There's that boss who was always so kind and patient with me. There's Ruffles. There's Fluffy. There's the lady who sang contralto in the choir. There's that nice old man I lived beside back when I was in high school. There's Hubby. Oh, how I miss him!"

We have to hunt through all these individual folders to find out where best to put this latest "grief" of ours. This latest triggering.

Pretty much all of this is done subconsciously, of course. But whether subconsciously or consciously, we re-experience every single "file" in there. And we subconsciously refile them over and over each time we must open that particular drawer.

It will be the same when we go through all the extra bowls at the back of the bottom shelf. It won't be easy. But it must be done.

Shouldn't Decluttering Be Called Ripping out My Soul?

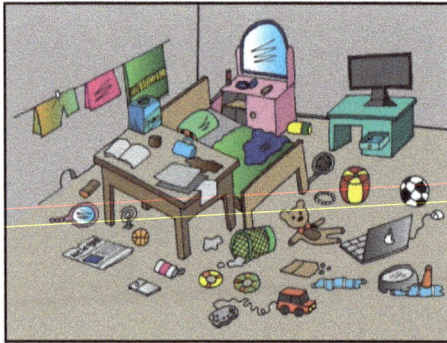

"My place is a mess with all this stuff lying around. Stuff I don't even..."

WHAT AM I DOING WITH ALL this stuff? Stuff I think I want but don't use. Some of it I'd even forgotten about.

I don't need even half of it. Not even a quarter of it. Maybe none.

Aha. What I'll do is move some of it out to the garage. Maybe rent a storage facility. Maybe put it all in the...

No. I'll still have the responsibility of it, won't I?

I have to rehome it.

But how?

How Indeed?

Let's get hold of three boxes or containers. Big ones.

We will label them:

1. KEEP
2. TOSS
3. DONATE

Let's think this through before we start:

"Toss" is a euphemism for "goes in the garbage."

The "KEEP" box will later be divided into (1) hand down to kids(s)/whomever; (2) keep (because I *need* it); and (3) dayum, I can't decide where this one goes.

Suggestions for the DONATE Box

Special stores in almost every community now sell used household goods and clothing that people have donated. The Salvation Army is only one. Any synagogue/ church/mosque will gladly act as go between for getting household goods to those in need of them. There are donation boxes specifically for clothing here and there in most cities and towns.

One of the lesser-realized places to donate things— anything—is to women's shelters. Many of these women have nothing but the clothes on their backs, literally, when they arrive at one of these shelters. (I was luckier.* Much luckier. In many, many ways.)

When I was in the women's shelter back in 2005, the house I was in would often call us down to the office to announce that someone had just donated a box of items. During my six weeks there, I was able to get started with the basics: a set of ancient Corelle dishes, for one. They also took us to a special clothing store where I got a winter coat.

These items were anything from blankets to spatulas. Things we never realize we *need* until we open the kitchen drawer in our new digs expecting, out of habit, to find one. (I still have the blanket. A comforter. A comforter in more ways than one.)

Men and women in halfway houses also need pretty much every single thing all of us old ladies have doubles and triples of, too. Do we actually *use* all those sheets and pillowcases from when the kids had bunk beds? How long ago was *that*?

----

*When I left my situation, I was lucky enough to be able to get some of my stuff into storage. My hundreds of books for one. But not much of my hundreds of dollars' worth of kitchen equipment and other things that I had brought into the situation in the first place (like a bed). Something to sleep on (my couch doubled as sofa and bed for quite some time) was more important than a mixer or a blender. That donated spatula was appreciated to no end. Books? With the advent of the Internet, I was able to rehome nearly all of the books I had been using as reference. materials.

Donating is a bonus in all directions. They get to start stocking their new residences. We get to help them do that. Nothing in good condition needs to go to waste.

How?

Right now, let's choose a cupboard shelf or a drawer we hardly ever go into and let's just get at it.

One shelf or one drawer to start. This has to be a pleasant first time. Do one. Stop. I repeat: Do one. Stop. Why? Psychologically, when we stop in the middle of something we like doing, or before we get tired, we want to get back to it as soon as possible. Like, tomorrow first thing.

Set up the boxes close by and sit on the floor. (I don't have trouble sitting on the floor, it's trying to get back up that's an issue. But this, too, can be accomplished with determination and mostly the will to survive.)

Using your own determination and will, take everything out of that drawer or off that shelf and put each thing into its respective box: KEEP, TOSS, DONATE.

Get yourself up off the floor. Grab a garbage bag. (You know exactly where you put those last time, right?)

Empty the TOSS box into it. Try to do this with neither regret nor flinching. Tie the top of the garbage bag and immediately march with pride to the garbage chute or garbage pail and let it slip from your fingers.

You did it! Woohoo. Yay!

Everything in the KEEP box goes back into that first drawer or onto that first shelf. (Bear with me.)

We will do nothing with the DONATE box right now.

Close the lids on the three boxes and stack them up somewhere for the next time. Tomorrow. Yes? First thing.

Walk away and forget about them. Go watch TV. Have a tea. Go for a walk.

"Tomorrow" Has Arrived

Get into position next to the second shelf (or drawer) and put everything there into its respective boxes.

The TOSS box gets emptied into another garbage bag and taken out. Immediately, right?

This time, the KEEP box's contents get put onto the **_first_** shelf/drawer with yesterday's things. There's room now, isn't there?

The DONATE box is starting to fill up.

The second shelf is empty. No kidding!

We will keep going like this until we've gone through every bureau/dresser/cupboard in our home.

When the first original shelf is full, start to fill up the second one. Then the third, etc.

We will keep using this same cupboard until all its shelves are full of our KEEP stuff. We'll deal with it soon, don't worry. We haven't been using any of this stuff anyway, have we?

Each time the DONATE box gets _full_, we will donate its contents and start filling it again.

It won't be long before our original bureau/dresser/cupboard is full but by then, we'll probably have another bureau/dresser/cupboard empty. Start filling up its drawers now. One at a time only!

Eventually, we'll realize that we have empty furniture

and cupboards and storage units all over the place.

We'll also realize that we have accomplished an amazing feat. We have decluttered our home from objects we didn't need, use or want anymore and we have probably made some woman or man's life easier by doing it. Our own, for one.

Let's start over with the first shelf that contains our KEEPs.

We will re-label the three boxes:
1. KIDS/EQUIVALENT
2. NEED
3. DECIDE

Using the same technique, we will go through everything again.

We will decide also, where our extra bureaus and bookcases will be going. We definitely need some of these. Yes, we do. But not all. This is another set of keep, toss, donate decisions.

Let's organize what's left using logic. If we don't know where everything is, what was the point of doing all this work in the first place? And from now on, we will put everything back where we got it from immediately after we use it. *Immediately after* we use it.

We're done!

Look at all the room I have. I can even dance around or do my Tai Chi without smashing my knee or my little toe on anything.

I have reorganized all my shelves and drawers and bookcases and I know exactly where everything is. I have just accomplished something impossibly amazing.

DISCLAIMER: This post is not intended to address hoarding. Hoarding requires professional attention. Hoarding is caused by as many reasons as there are hoarders.

Now What?

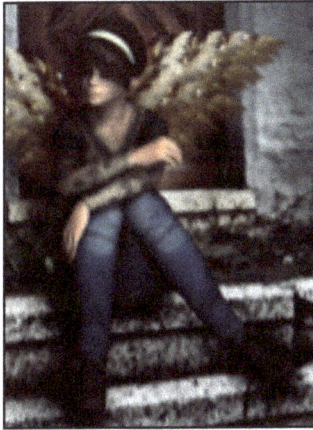

"I have nothing to live for. I am of no value to anyone."

L IFE AS I'VE ALWAYS KNOWN IT is no longer. I'm useless. I'm bored. I'm lost. I'm depressed. I have no value. If I can't be someone's 3C*, what good am I?

Before Women's Liberation, certain things were expected of females. We were trained to not just act a certain way, but to be and to think a certain way. If we refused to conform, we could not ever expect to get a good

---

*The definition of a "3C" will be revealed in a future post. It's rude and possibly shocking. But sadly apt.

husband. Or even a bad one. And all women were required to have a husband. Men needed wives, after all. They were out there working, making money, spending free time with their fellows to recharge, ruling the world, making important decisions. And there we were, all trained and smiling, full of hope while we waited. Me, hoping they wouldn't notice my small breasts, my tall stature or my attitude of "but how come boys don't have to do all this sh*t, too?"

Females were trained to cook and clean. Even in [most] homes in the old days when almost every home had a servant, the "lady of the house" had to know how to cook and clean so she would know what to expect from her servants. (I see on one branch of my own family tree, about five generations back, that one family of servants had servants, too.)

Let's say someone is trained to do a specific task and for some reason, that task becomes redundant. They lose their job, their career, their purpose. They can plunge themselves into the darkness of depression and despair believing they are no longer of value. Or they can learn something new and do that.

Women of my generation were raised with one basic purpose in mind: to be a wife.

What is a wife?

Let me rephrase that: What *was* a wife? Things have changed! (Somewhat.)

During WWII (World War Two, 1939–1945), men went off to war and women stepped into their vacated jobs. Remember Rosie the Riveter (https://www.history.com/topics/world-war-ii/rosie-the-riveter) That was what our moms did. That was what women were capable of doing.

When the war was over, the men came home and got their jobs back and...

Where did the women go? The women who had been "working?"

They went home to do what they were "created for."

Single women were "allowed" to be in the workforce as secretaries, teachers, nurses and librarians, but as soon as that ring went on that finger... Pow. Zapped into the world of the 3C, the world of The Wife.

Women didn't "work," women were housewives. That wasn't work. The natural state of the female was to be at home. Women loved it. They loved looking after the house and the kids and their husbands. ("And they lived happily ever after.")

Remember what I said above? "They lose their job, their career, their purpose. They can plunge themselves into the darkness of depression and despair believing they are no longer of value. Or they can learn something new and do that."

My mother was in the Royal Canadian Air Force during WWII. She worked as a telephone operator. She married my father who was also in the RCAF. (Dad trained wireless operators.) She was now a wife.

Mom did her wifely duties, of course she did. But she could also sew. Like a boss. She made my clothes and her own. She did my hair. She was wife, nurse, teacher, fashion designer, hair stylist, chef-ette and often a single mom when Dad was away, still in the Air Force, then sick in the hospital for two months with a form of typhoid fever, then away at police school when I was around five. She did it all. That's what women did.

What else was there to do? There were no cell phones. No TV. No microwaves. Not everyone had a telephone. Many in the boonies didn't even have electricity. I remember visiting a cousin's farm in the 1950s and they had these big glass lamps that they lit at night. No electricity. On a dairy farm.

Post-war times were tough. Mom had a washboard to do the laundry with until 1950. This I remember well because I got sh*t for blabbing to the mailman when he knocked on our apartment door one day: "We got a washing machine because Mommy is going to have a baby." Pregnancy in those days was generally kept secret because there was only one way to get into that condition.

What Did a Wife Do in Those Days?

What occupations kept "the wife" occupied during those long, long days of being all alone in the house while her beloved, her prince, was away at work? What did she do all day to "fill in her time?"

She:
- cooked and baked (Despite the idea that girls "didn't need to know" arithmetic in school, our mothers could double, triple, halve and even third any recipe without the use of an abacus. There were no electronic calculators back then.)
- cleaned (This, with mop and pail, watered-down vinegar for windows (Dad did the outside

of the windows), and cloths that had to be washed. There were no [affordable] vacuum cleaners, paper towels (as we know them) or "magic" sponges in those days. Floors were washed on hands and knees. The latter I know from experience!)

- did the laundry (Mom and most moms I knew of did the laundry on Mondays in a wringer washer. Watch your fingers! Clothes were hung on the line no matter the weather, although we did have a folding wooden rack of sorts for emergencies.)

- ironed (Pretty much every single thing that went through the washing machine—dish towels, sheets, pillowcases, Hubby's undershorts—was ironed. And this was a Tuesday job. Imagine irons without electricity! https://www.pressrepublican.com/news/lifestyles/ironing-more-tedious-with-sad-irons/article_d5c1a6fe-749d-5eb2-a87a-a8400cac347e.html)

- served as escort for public events with Hubby (Including all that that implies. [*wink, wink*])

- "babysat"

- home schooled (Helped with the homework. But Daddy was often called in for the arithmetic. (See above).)

- made sure the children and hubby were fed, dressed and out the door on time for school, work and religious services

- handled phone calls (In those post-war days, in our town, there were party lines or sometimes the neighbor's phone if families didn't have a phone yet.)
- acted as doctor and nurse (Doctors made house calls and charged money for it, money people didn't often have, so our mothers had to know all about mustard plasters, Mercurochrome, iodine, ice packs, a little gin for bad colds, how to take a sliver out or a bee's stinger, diagnose when to actually call in a doctor; name it, she could do it.)
- shopped (within an extremely strict budget that usually Hubby was in charge of; girls didn't know anything about arithmetic, right?)
- dressed to the nines (especially in time for Hubby's arrival for supper which was ALWAYS on the table when he stepped through the doorway)
- had the newspaper and radio all ready for Hubby after supper so he could relax after his hard day at work
- kept the children occupied in the evenings so Hubby wouldn't be disturbed (All this while doing the dishes and helping the kids do their homework (see above) and later, getting them ready for bed. Then be all glamorous and spiffed-up (see "escort" above) to spend time with Hubby after the kids were taken care of.)
- I could go on and on and on

"Imagine, if you will..." this wife having none of this to do anymore. No kids, no hubby, a vacuum cleaner (maybe even a Roomba, too), a microwave, restaurants for take-out, order from or dine in, a cell phone with reminders, TV that can be recorded then watched whenever, drug-stores, OHIP (Ontario Health Insurance Plan) or equivalent (in most countries), mixers, blenders, juicers, frozen pre-made meals, prepared almost-everything, refrigerators, freezers, washing machines and dryers, debit and credit cards, a job/career/government pension that provides a stable income, pre-school, daycare, a car...

Wow. Nothing to do. I'm of no value anymore. "They lose their job, their career, their purpose. They can plunge themselves into the darkness of depression and despair believing they are no longer of value. Or they can learn something new and do that."

It's never too late to learn something new. Some-thing fun. Volunteer. Take an online course or go back to school/college/university. Write a book. Write two. Think of something. We now have 31,536,000 seconds a year to ourselves.

Three... Two... One.
[*gunshot*]

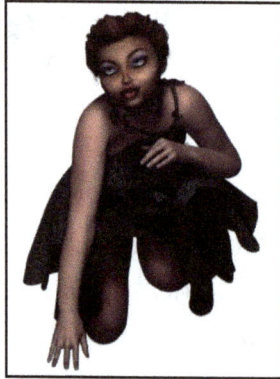

"Wait! What? I was never trained for this!"

WHAT ARE YOU TALKING ABOUT, TELLING me to get out there and do something new?

We old ladies don't know how to do anything other than what we've always done. We aren't supposed to be doing anything other than what we were trained for, created for, meant for. Right?

No, no, no. Doing something new is way too scary.

And isn't it kind of "forbidden" or something?

Aren't we supposed to carry on like always? Even though that "always" has changed so very much for us? Even though we've emptied our home of everything we don't need and have no family around to do things for, we old ladies don't know how to do anything other than what we've always done.

No, no, no.

Besides, if we do anything "different," all the old ladies in our community will tsk tsk us so much, their dentures will come flying out. Haven't we always "obeyed" our elders?

Wait! What? We're the elders now. What are we doing being terrified of all those old tongues (and dentures)?

Hmm. Maybe... Doing something we've never done might be worth a thought. It might even be... fun?

How about we take it one step at a time? Ease into it?

How about we take our training and experiences and knowledge into the world outside our cave and massage it into something the real world needs?

In future posts, I'll go into more detail about Things We Old Ladies Can Do outside the Home, but for now, here are some thoughts that might help transition us from the concept of always doing what's expected of us, to doing what's unexpected.

Things have gotten better and better and better. Of course, they have. Men today do housework and do it well. They sometimes work from home while their wives go out to work, and this includes cooking, cleaning and "baby-sitting." Nobody (generally, right?) seems to care anymore who does what in the home.

But...

I'm talking about us old gals in this blog. We—and

our men—were programmed much differently. And a lot more strongly, it seems.

One Warning

I really hesitate to say anything about this as I don't want readers to think I'm anti-having-a-husband/boyfriend. I'm not. I'm speaking of (generally) North America because that's where I live and where my parents were born and grew up, and where three of my grandparents were born and grew up.

But... Here's the advice.

Don't jump into a new relationship just yet.

Wait a while.

Wait as though you're involved in a drug or alcohol rehab program where they recommend not being in a relationship with anyone for at least a year of sobriety.

Why?

If we do get involved, we'll never learn anything new. We'll never "escape" from the notion that we are of no value being other than a 3C.

Men of "our generation" have been very strongly programmed toward the 3C woman just as much as we have, and it seems that nothing can alter their programmed view.

Our fathers were involved in WWII whether they served or not. When the war was over, women went back home. The only way to do this, to get women to go back home and let the men take the jobs again, was through propaganda. Propaganda aimed at both men and women. Movies were a huge part of this propaganda. (Yes they were!)

But it goes back much, much further than that and the trouble started when "man" became "civilized."

What Am I Talking About?

I'm talking about the switch from caveman—er, sorry, I mean caveperson—to royalty. And apparently, we didn't really live in caves, we were nomads, we lived where we could: https://en.wikipedia.org/wiki/Caveman

In the days of the caveperson, the females would have had children hanging off them or inside them or both, so would not always be nimble enough to dodge the hooves, horns, tusks, teeth or beaks of potential food. So generally—*generally*—the males were the hunters. The task of gathering would fall—generally—to the females. (Is this when we developed our shopping skills? Or lack thereof?)

These roles reversed when required. If not, *Homo sapiens* would have gone extinct. All members of the group shared their experiences, their knowledge, their abilities. And this is where storytelling began, too:

"You should have seen the look on your husband's face when that mammoth turned around and started running in his direction." General laughter all around the campfire.

And because the women did most of the gathering, they did most of the tasting and testing of berries and plants. The women, then, became the scientists, the doctors, but they shared this information with daughters and sons alike; and with the older men who no longer hunted for whatever reason.

The men, the hunters, would have developed an amazing ability to get back home no matter what. That's right, they didn't need to read directions. That skill has been retained. And it's an innate skill, not something to be made fun of.

Everyone in the entire group was equal. Even the children were listened to with respect.

Then "civilization" came along and equality was gone with the wind.

Civilization:
The Ruination of "Humanity" in Humans

Civilization meant staying in one place to tend to the crops.

Crops meant owning land.

Owning land meant protecting land.

Protecting land meant killing anybody trying to take it from you.

Oops.

Once again the men were away, but this time, they were away trying to get their land back. Or, in some cases, take over someone else's land because they didn't have any or they needed more because their families were growing.

They were impregnating other women and men were impregnating our women.

Women no longer "gathered" so were no longer the healers, the scientists.

And while the men were away killing people and taking back (taking over?) as much land as they could, they needed someone to take care of the crops for them so they either hired people or captured people (the beginnings of slavery?) to do that.

The person (man) who "owned" the most land was now the most powerful in the region. He'd killed so many people on the way "up," everyone was afraid of him. And wisely so.

He would allow people to use parts of his land in exchange for either goods or "money." People paid him. (Um. Would this have been referred to as "rent?" Or as "tax?") These people were grateful to be safe and protected on *his* land and to be able to eke out a living there. He had become wealthy from the spoils of war, the "rent" from *his* property, and the sale of *his* wheat. He had complete control. He became ruler. King.

His son would take over from him. Had to be *his* son so "the wife" was watched carefully so as not to be impregnated by anyone else. (Women were regarded as incubators of the man's seed.) Rules came about regarding what a woman could and could not do. What a woman should and should not do.

Men took over and any man who disagreed with the king's rules (= laws of the land now) was executed. Good motivation to go along with the current views of society, eh?

The new land became a country ruled by its king.

Then along came the king's advisor who could go by many names: soothsayer, wizard, diviner, prophet, religious figure... And this man—yes, a man—made all the rules for men and women alike. And this, as you know, has stuck like Gorilla Glue for millennia. (When I was in Chichen Itza several years ago, our tour guide told us that it was not the Spanish who ruined the Maya civilization, it was the soothsayer. This soothsayer had "mis-soothed" and an entire civilization went down the tubes.)

So let's not blame "our men" for turning us into 3Cs. It's been going on for a long, long time. When I think of the men of my generation, I picture the kids I hung out with in the double-dead-end-streets section of my small home town.

The young boys were the sons of fathers who'd served in WWII. (See above re fighting to maintain one's land from those trying to take it from us.) Some of the fathers had been killed. Some of the fathers were "shell shocked," today's equivalent of PTSD (Post Traumatic Stress Disorder). The father of my own best friend in the neighborhood had been shot down in the Netherlands when she was in utero.

These boys had learned from their fathers, fathers who were dead or alive or suffering from a mental disorder, to always be protective, even unto death. It was their duty to protect, especially to protect their women—called "girls" in those days. (The word "woman" back then bore the connotation of non-virgin. Tsk, tsk.)

The boys in my 'hood grew up with this idea firmly entrenched in their psyches. And so did the "girls."

We've been trained—programmed!—to be and think and act a certain way.

Is it not time for a change? To take a leap of faith that we won't crash and burn if we do something for ourselves for a change?

————

Reference: *The Murderer Next Door: Why the Mind is Designed to Kill* https://www.amazon.ca/Murderer-Next-Door-Mind-Designed-ebook/dp/B002IEUVBY/ref=sr_1_1?dchild=1&keywords=the+murderer+next+door&qid=1619783861&sr=8-1

I'm Ready to Evolve!
Let's Do Something
Different!

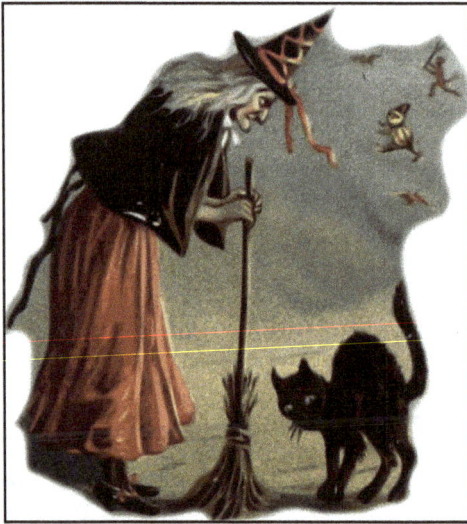

"Think of it as a decompression chamber between lives."

ONE THING WE OLD LADIES CAN volunteer for is fostering for animal rescue groups.

(It's not only dogs that require fostering. There are rescue groups for cats and other critters as well.)

Many families had at least one dog (or kitty). If we

had good luck with these critters, meaning we treated them like family and took them to training classes and regular veterinary appointments, we could offer our services to a dog-rescue group for fostering.

NOTE: Foster homes are not the easiest for rescue groups to find so we must control ourselves and relinquish the wee adorable darlings when the time comes to surrender them to their forever homes. We must be strong. Another foster will come along.

Besides, we are now "elderly." What happens if we decide to keep this critter and we suddenly end up in long-term care? What happens to the critter? Off it goes to a foster home until a forever home comes along? The exact same reason, in some cases, we would be fostering this wee dolly in the first place?

When my kitty crossed the rainbow bridge a few years ago, friends were astonished that I didn't try to replace him. Not that he *could* be replaced, Bixby was unique.

Here he is as Mieuw Heffner.

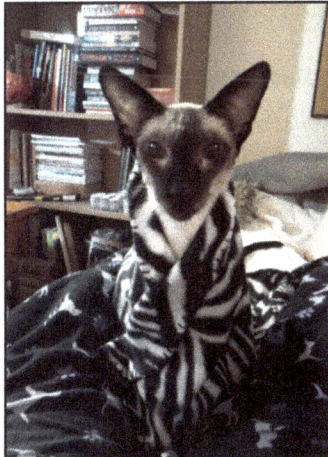

And here he is audition-posing in case somebody starts up a *Playkitty Magazine.*

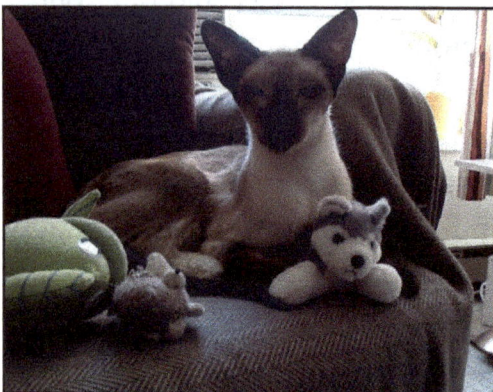

Yes. Bixby was a ham, among other things. When I was showing and breeding Rottweilers in another life, he was my good-cop puppy trainer. (His Auntie Zest was bad cop.*) Bixby came from a show-cat home, so I think that's why he liked dressing up and getting his picture taken. He was used to being handled and used to the limelight. I missed him like crazy, but...

---

*I remember one particular "recess" for one of my litters when everybody was running around in the living room, raising hell (essentially learning how to go potty on the paper). Bixby was right in the middle of it all. Not so his Auntie Zest. Zest had disappeared into the kitchen. I noticed that one by one, the puppies seemed to go into the kitchen and go out of sight there. Within seconds, I would hear a *yike*, then the puppy would run full tilt back to his buddies, probably yelling, "Shiiiiiiiiiiiiiiiiiiit! I'm never going anywhere NEAR that thing again!"

My thinking was that if a "replacement" kitty lived for sixteen years as Bixby had done, that would put me very close to 90 by then. What if the "replacement" kitty lived until it was twenty? Twenty-one? Twenty-two? Would I still be alive? My sight is going, my hearing is going. Could I care properly for a by-then-aging-too kitty? Nope. It wouldn't be fair to bring a new kitty into my life permanently.

Fostering is a noble act of love.

What's Involved in Fostering?

How does this blog writer know about animal-rescue groups and fostering in the first place? I do volunteer administrative work for a local dog rescue group, and have done so for years.

A friend of mine fosters for another Ottawa area dog-rescue group.

To foster, we need to have sufficient knowledge and experience with said species. Many of these animals come from horrendous conditions and need compassionate, experienced, patient, knowledgeable people to help them transition from Hell to new home.

(When I say "horrendous conditions," I will only tell you that I worked for an emergency veterinary hospital as a receptionist for four years in the early 1990s. I tell people, now, that I saw things there that I would not put into the head of my worst enemy. So don't ask.)

Foster parents need the ability to evaluate the critters in their care to help the rescue group decide the kind of forever home it would be best suited for. Would this particular dog get along with other dogs, with cats, with children? What age could children be or not be? Same thing for cats.

The group I volunteer for provides food, veterinary care, toys, collars and leashes and beds and anything else a foster dog requires. All that would be required from you is your kindness and expertise.

Perhaps we're in a situation where we would like to do something to help out critter-rescue groups but for whatever reason, we aren't able to house one to foster it. (I'm in that situation.) Or perhaps our experience/knowledge is not vast enough for the rescue group to allow one of their charges to be fostered by us. (Yet?)

If we have a vehicle, we can do something else wonderful. We can offer to drive a rescued animal from one location to another.

These "drives" work on a "relay system" and are an amazing way to get an animal from point A to point Z without any individual driver spending more than perhaps an hour or two (including their trip back home), but the animal ends up being transported for perhaps hundreds of miles.

I sat shotgun when a friend did this several years ago. It feels good. Really good. Those who are less experienced with animal behavior might consider riding shotgun until they learn more.

NOTE: Be sure to do background research before you jump into contacting a local rescue group, though. Most are well-intentioned. Most. Almost all of them, in fact. Find someone who does volunteer work for each of the groups in your area, approach them and ask for their opinion of the other groups. Ask several. Then decide for yourself.

The Gift of Your Experience Can Make Lives Better

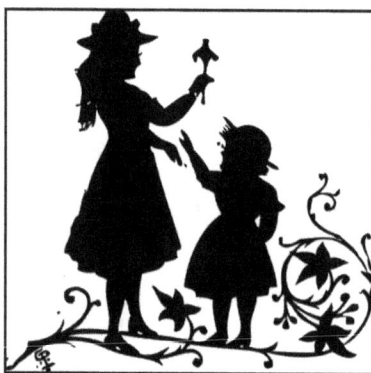

"And this is how we can make that happen. See how it works?"

When I did an online search for "senior" and "volunteer," I came up with an amazing number of projects and programs that seniors—both women and men—can get involved in. My search generated actual organizations throughout the USA and Canada but I won't list individual contact information here. For example, the Canadian projects and programs I found are mostly centered in Toronto but I'm certain every city or town or village has something along these lines. If they don't, why not start one?

I will list what I found with a brief synopsis for those that had synopses to synopsize. (Can't do the actual copy/paste of what they posted because of copyright.)

I recommend contacting the City/Town/Village Hall in your area to see what they are offering. There are also Community Centers that, I'm certain, would welcome volunteers of any age.

Deep Breath!

Best way to do all this searching and contacting is, of course, by using a computer.

Nooooo!

Yeeeees!

Now that we have whittled down our "busy" lives to have time for ourselves, we don't want to spend all that time on hold. Do we! No we don't! We aren't going to spend hours on the telephone now, are we! No we aren't!

I hope my next post will alleviate some of the abject terror females of our generation seem to harbor about computers; as well as the crazy idea that "girls" are too stupid to be able to operate one, with or without efficiency.

Now, off we go into the wild, blue yonder of the volunteer world.

Volunteer with Children, Teach, Coach Sports

Whatever we learned along the way about sports, either from what our own children learned in school—and rubbed off on us—or from what we ourselves learned doing our own thing, is more than some kids know when starting out. Think about it. We can help, if only to encourage.

Construction Volunteering

This is something I never in my wildest dreams would have thought about doing even though I am inclined that way. It's a rare occasion when I have to call in the troops to help out with any projects in my home, so yes, I know how to wield a hammer. I'm sure most of us old ladies do. If not, we can learn. Right? At least we could hand out lemonade to the workers.

Women's Empowerment Volunteering

Maybe this is what I'm doing with this blog? Attempting to "empower" us old ladies to get out there and believe in ourselves again? Like we were allowed to do pre-puberty? Before all the "rules of society" kicked in to smother our spirit? I'm sure we know how to empower younger women to do this, so I'd say, all we need is practice. When we teach, we learn too.

Public Health Volunteering

Once again, contact City/Town/Village Hall to see what programs they have.

Wildlife Conservation Volunteering

This can involve walks in the bush, birdwatching, photography... Or even learning *how* to walk in the bush, birdwatch and photograph wildlife in the first place.

Marine Conservation Volunteering

This involves diving. Those who've gone traveling and went on a scuba jaunt will know what's involved here. I don't. I'm not a traveler. However, when I would attend girls camp every summer as a kid, I loved to swim underwater. It was more interesting under there. And I could cover a lot of "ground" because I have big feet that doubled as flippers.

We can help with coral reef conservation research and marine plastic pollution prevention by getting involved with something like this. (I saw a TV program about this a few weeks ago, so it looks like it's getting to be a "thing.")

Other Ideas

Collecting, serving, preparing, or distributing food.
Fundraising or selling items to raise money.
Driving seniors to appointments.
Engaging in general labor, like helping build homes or clean up parks.
Tutoring or teaching.
Mentoring the youth.
Collecting, making, or distributing clothing.
Writing that book.

Canadian Assoc.. for Retired Persons (CARP)

From what I understand, this is a lobby group. Or, at least, a group that lobbies? According to the posted blurb, there are 26 chapters across Canada that focus on "improving health care and financial security for aging Canadians."

Other Ideas

These are mostly Toronto-based but we can approach our own City/Town/Village Hall to see if anything similar is available.

Native Canadian Centre of Toronto (NCCT)
Special Olympics Ontario
Nanny Angel Network
Girls Inc. York Region

More Suggestions I Found Online

See caution note below.

Act globally.
Be a foster grandparent.
Volunteer at a national park.
Lend a hand at your local library.
Run, walk or cycle for a good cause.
Walk dogs (Humane Society and SPCA, etc.).
Join the Peace Corps.
Become an activist.
Assist older citizens. (I guess this would be citizens our age? Younger?)
Provide a hot meal.
Help out at a favorite museum.
Volunteer virtually.
Organize your own fundraiser.

Join a mosque/church/synagogue group, a choir.
Work at shelters to hand out food.
Cook for shelters if you're good at mass producing.
Work at a hospital "store."

How to Find out What's Available?

As I said, the best way for finding out many things these days, is, of course, with a computer search. I hope my next post will ease some of the fears associated with using computers.

A Note of Caution

When we were born, the population of the world was... Oh, wait. They jumped from 1927 (at 2,000,000,000, which looks like a guestimate to me) to 1951. There are no data for the years between 1927 and 1951. For 1951, the world population is listed as 2,584,034, 261. The world population for 2020 is listed as 7,794,798,739.

("Source: Worldometer (www.Worldometers.info) From 1950 to current year: Elaboration of data by United Nations, Department of Economic and Social Affairs, Population Division. World Population Prospects: The 2019 Revision. (Medium-fertility variant).")

This means:
- there are about 5 billion more Earthlings looking for ways to make a living;
- there are many of these who will do just about anything to make that happen.

Not everyone on planet Earth is bad; not everyone

on planet Earth is good.

Bottom line? When you find a group to volunteer your valuable services with, double check with the authorities to ensure they are legit and not some female (or male, either) sex-trafficking outfit, or a fake baby adoption center, a group that goes out there collecting people's organs, or a drug cartel. Yes, these groups exist. But so do the good ones.

The Computer: The Bane of Us Old Ladies? (Part I)

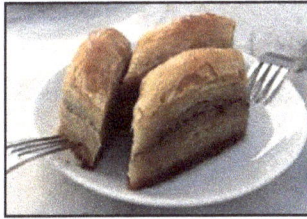

"Easy as pie?" More like, easy as baklava.
(In two parts. I got carried away.)

MANY WOMEN IN MY GENERATION HAVE this idea that computers are monstrous creatures who say things like, "I'm sorry, Dave. I'm afraid I can't do that." (Hal, *2001: A Space Odyssey*)

And we don't yet have robots like Robby from the 1956 *Forbidden Planet*. At least, not affordable ones. Not yet. Although... I do have a Roomba. His name is Cecil. The one who washes the floor is Brendan.

I have an "Alexa," too. She's really great. She helps me spell things; she tells me the weather. She'll play a radio station. She plays music. She will read (not well, though) any e-books I've purchased from Amazon. When I'm watching TV and am nice and comfy on the sofa, instead of getting up (while yelling "ow, ow") and heading for my computer to check out something somebody just said in a program, I ask her. Sometimes, however, she says "I'm sorry. I don't know that." (I would really like it if she could say that kind of thing in Hal's voice. And call me "Dave.")

So computers are great things to have.

What's so dangerous about them then? Was hubby lying when he told us to be afraid, be very afraid?

No he wasn't, but...

Have a look at what *might* come up when we search for something.

I had searched for "wordpress." (Without the quotation marks. And there's no need to capitalize words when searching. Usually.)

(See opposite page.)

Take a look at the small print in the top line of each item. Beside "Ad." (The smallest print.) The *fourth* one is the actual WordPress.com site I was wanting because it says https://wordpress.com and nothing else. The others would not have led me to where I wanted to go.

The others (and they vary each search) are hoping for business. The others are hoping we'll "accidentally" click on them and "buy" *their* wares instead. These are not necessarily "evil" companies, they're just hoping. But some *ARE* "evil," so be careful. Think of the old days when we were warned not to accept candy from strangers.

Bottom line? Be absolutely certain that the site you are clicking on is the one you are looking for. Yes, yes, I know. I am instilling paranoia into my readers again, but once you get used to doing all this, you will gain confidence. So do the "bad guys," too, though. Just be aware.

Don't be paranoid, be wary. Study. Learn. Ask. Think of it as a game you're playing against the "enemy." Be like

James Bond and thwart the dairty boogers.

Here's a link to an interesting take on antivirus programs: https://en.softonic.com/articles/3-dirty-tricks-that-antivirus-companies-dont-want-you-to-know-about? utm_source=softonic&utm_medium=email&utm_campaig n=nl_w21&utm_source=Softonic&utm_campaign=e2e44b be34-EMAIL_CAMPAIGN_5_25_2020_21_38_COPY_01& utm_medium=email&utm_term=0_9576753237- e2e44bbe34-210745910

(My apologies for such a long, complicated link that you would need to actually type out since this is a print book, but, if you have nothing to do for the next... let's say... half an hour? Give it a shot. But I recommend typing it into a Word file first; proofread it; then copy/paste. It has to be *exact*, eh?)

I say "an interesting take" because I copied all that big, long stream to ensure it would lead to where it said it would go (for my blog peeps' sakes). Then when I pasted it into my browser to see it, all kinds of ads kept leaping in while I was scrolling down. The very thing the article told me some antivirus programs would do to me.

You will note that the main "dude" is Softonic dot com. I "heard" they are notorious for following us around and throwing ads at us. Perhaps it's true? About them, I mean. That said, the article is very close to what I am recommending. So thank you, Softonic. [*kiss hug kiss*] (And I've used programs from Softonic.)

When there are ads tossed in here and there at sites you visit, check the corners of the ads' boxes—usually the upper right corner—to see if there's an X there. If so, click on it and that ad will disappear. Hopefully forever. (This X can be in other corners, too. They're starting to *hide* them. Bastids!) Some of them are like flypaper though.

You will also have legitimate-looking and actually legitimate things pop in, too. They will ask us to click Yes or No. X those.

Yup. "They're coming to get you, Barbara."*

Why Am I So Afraid of Computers?

What will happen if I click on something *wrong*†? Will the computer explode? No. (Although that does happen in some TV shows like *Criminal Minds, et al.*)

What exactly is so scary about computers? On its own, a computer is essentially a glorified electric typewriter.

Is it the computer itself we fear then?

On its own, no, but when it's connected to the Internet, it morphs into a kind of telegraph machine. (These work on radio frequencies.) And it works both ways: sending information to us and from us. Sometimes, whether we know it or not.

So is it the Internet we should fear then?

---

*1968, *Night of the Living Dead*.

†Years ago, I belonged to a New Age group. A teacher spoke one evening about using the words, "right and wrong." She recommended we stop doing that as it was self-judging in a negative way most of the time. She said we might consider using "right and not right."

No. That would be like being afraid of a lamp cord that was just sitting there passing electrons through to the lamp's lightbulb.

What should we be afraid of about computers then?

Why do we lock our doors at night? It's not against the dark. It's against the possibility of humans gaining access to our home and either stealing from us or doing us harm when it's dark.

So. It's not the computer we should be afraid of and it's not the Internet.

Exactly. It's not the computer that's at fault.

It's humans. Most humans are kind and trusting. Some humans are mean.

Danger Lurks

Back to *Criminal Minds* again: There are those who, through the Internet, lure children, teenagers and naïve adults into meeting them, then cause them great harm. (Online, women are more likely to be targets because we are perceived to be "weak" and "stupid.")

Think about this though:

We would actually have to meet this person in real life, or give "him" (usually a male—usually!) our home address for anything dangerous to happen to us physically. So that's not the computer's fault, that's our own fault for trusting someone when we shouldn't. Be wary of psychopaths in wolves' clothing who are offering us candy both on the physical street and online.

And while I think of it, if your computer is newish, it will probably have a little pinhole up along the top edge, the "rim" around the screen, probably near the center. See it there? This is a camera. Snip off a little square of duct tape and cover this pinhole over. I had heard about this but thought I was perhaps being a tad paranoid, but I asked my IT guy his thoughts and he said, very quietly,

"Yes. Cover it."

It's Mostly Monetary Harm that Can Befall Us

What will happen if we get cyber-attacked? Hacked. Or if we hit a button we shouldn't?

It's gonna cost us money. Bottom line. *Money.* Somebody once said, "Economics is everything." (I think that statement gets truer and truer these days.)

Hackers and cyber bullies can climb in through your computer's windows, its attic, through its basement by digging a tunnel... We need alarms set up everywhere. But we don't need to be sitting at the window with binoculars. We need reliable, trustworthy bodyguards.

NOTE: I'm not referring to the Windows program (capital "W"), I'm trying to make a comparison about how "they" can invade our computers, comparing it to how burglars might invade our homes. Example: There's a virus referred to as a Trojan and it works like a Trojan horse. It sneaks in and hides "in the basement" or "in the attic." Talk to an IT expert about this.

The IT expert will tell us that the main thing is to get a good antivirus program. We will need to renew this (pay for it) perhaps yearly, semi-yearly, monthly...

We need to have an IT (Information Technology) expert set us up initially with an antivirus program s/he recommends. Information Technology experts cost money, too. It's usually an hourly rate.

My own programs, recommended by an IT guy, are from an online company that I've been using for nearly 15 years. It offers several (individual, separate) apps (apps = applications) that I pay for on an annual basis. They offer more, but these are the ones I need, so use.

1. antivirus protection
2. tune-up
3. driver updater
4. secure VPN

All of these are excellent protection against hackers. (Hackers are ***holes who have nothing better to do than try to make other people sad and angry, and/or poor and frustrated, and/or scared. They especially like to make us scared.)

I also use two apps (with semi-annual payments) that "hunt" for (1) "spies" and for (2) files that have "lost their way." (Sometimes our files can get bumped out of the way on the hard drive. Hard drive? The hard drive is the computer's brain. Think of a hard drive as being a super-duper long-playing record like we used to use in the old days. Remember those? With their grooves and the needle? The needle that could screech across our album if we weren't careful? Hard drives can and do "re-write" their "grooves" as we work on our computers. They can get "scratched," too. Hard drives hold thousands and thousands of "songs" on them, and sometimes things can get jiggled off track. The second program noted above helps repair issues.)

Regardless. We must perform regular maintenance. As in, weekly maintenance. But have your IT person show you how to do this. And take notes upon notes while s/he does this. And remember where you put these notes. (See previous post about putting things back where they were.) Or, pay your IT expert several hundred dollars a week to come in and do this for you. No? Learn to do basic, regular maintenance and follow through.

(I've heard that Apple/Mac computers don't need any of this maintenance or antivirus diligence. I don't know. I don't use Apple/Mac so can't advise. Ask your IT person.)

NOTE: Be careful not to remove "old Windows backup files" when doing maintenance. Don't remove "restore points" either. I am speaking from experience.

The Computer: The Bane of Us Old Ladies? (Part II)

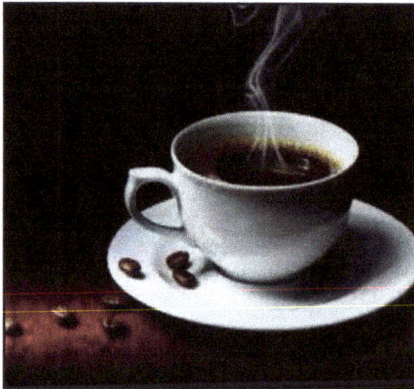

"Easy does it!"

When we are online, we tend not to blink as much. This is not good for anyone, especially those with dry eye syndrome. Something I learned when I was type-setting many years ago (i.e., spending eight hours a day plus, typing on a computer), was to look away often. Get up and go look out a window into the distance every now and again. Remember to blink. Close both eyes for several seconds to let them recoup.

Protect your NECK!

Because I write for myself and edit and design for other Indie writers, my go-to work station is my desktop computer. It's on a regular computer desk. I use a large monitor (screen) so I am basically looking straight ahead when I'm on it. (I was a typesetter for 20 years so I know how to type all day without negative effects. Not that I do, of course! My wrists and hands scream at me these days if I take advantage of them.)

I also have a laptop that I switch to, e.g., whenever maintenance is going on with my desktop, but since it sits on my coffee table, I can't be on it too long. Using a laptop on a coffee table makes us bend over and tilt our heads back. This affects our necks.

If I'm going to be using my laptop for any length of time, I use my special box to set it on. I used black Con-Tact® paper to wrap an ordinary, but sturdy, cardboard box. Color doesn't matter. I just liked the black. (That's my TV behind it. I listen to the radio on my TV while I work.)

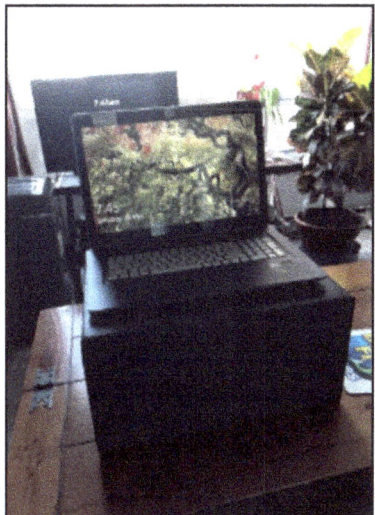

Ask

Ask your grandchildren or great grands to show you how to write an email.

By all means, bank online. No issue there. Just

make sure not to "save" your password; type it in every time. And, most important: **Ensure that you are on an actual bank's site when you sign up! And when you sign back in!** Maybe have your IT guy/gal show you some tricks for this, too.

I keep recommending "the IT guy/gal" and that's because they for certain know what they're doing. They went to school for it. Many of them went into debt to go to school for it. They know what they're doing. Many of our children and grands know what they're doing. I know what I'm doing—most of the time—because I was working on a computer in 1969. But when I run into issues, do I ask the next door neighbor's kid? No. I ask my IT guy.

Warning

DO NOT, DO NOT, DO NOT get sucked into those posts on Facebook (etc.) that ask you to click on your birth month, or pet's name, or anything that might even in the tiniest, slightest bit, reveal what your passwords could be.

This is how hackers can find out a lot of information about you. Information that can lead them to know your passwords, banking information, your mother's maiden name, and other information about you and your life.

I'm not going to tell you how to set up a password. In fact, when you set up your password, don't tell anybody how you set yours up, either. Most places now require that you use a capital letter, a number, a symbol, and maybe something else. Figure something out that can be changed on a regular basis in some way, but that you can easily remember.

When publicly online on Facebook and apps like it, assume there are hackers watching you. Because there are. I go on Facebook every day and really like it, but I'm aware.

Main thing is to get a good antivirus program and *know how to use it.*

When you begin to get comfortable with emailing, be extremely wary with incoming emails that:

- seem weird
- are from an unknown sender
- issue a threat (like, "Sorry to have to tell you this but we have hacked your computer." This message is pure shite! BUT! If you open that particular email and respond to it... Well, they warned you, right? You will have been hacked then.)

Do not open anything like this. I know it is tempting to "just peek" but that's how they get ya.

You will sometimes even get emails that appear to be from yourself. This is pure shite, too. DO NOT OPEN. Click on "Mark as Junk" (if you have that app) and carry on.

We often get emails that tell us about updates for the programs we run, for the banks we use, for this and for that.

Please notice that emails from your bank (e.g.) won't have an actual link to where you can open your bank account in that particular email. Some do. Most don't. They tell you to go there and find it at their actual site. NOT through an email link.

"Be afraid, be very afraid" of emails that contain links to your personal, sensitive, online accounts. Close the email and go to the source yourself.

More on Maintenance

When we are doing our maintenance, we need to include clearing out the "Inbox" and deleted files from our emailing app.

The way my emailing program works, I can right click on an email and it will give me a list that contains the command: "Mark as junk." I do, and off it goes into the Junk folder. (To be deleted later on.) NOTE: Not all emailing programs offer this feature.

I delete my deleted files and junk files about once a month or so. I get a LOT of emails. There's also the "Sent" folder, too, that needs deleting from. Those emails get deleted, too. (If I don't need to keep them. See below for how to organize that.)

I have noticed that some people tend to keep aaaaaalllll their emails in their Inbox. Yikes. Time to declutter!

What I have done is "create" folders that I can "move" dealt-with emails to. Like I mentioned in a previous post, we can get rid of what we don't want, and store everything else in "drawers" or on "shelves" so we'll know where they are at all times. (Ask your IT guy to demonstrate.)

Example: I have a folder for my family, one for my business, one for this, one for that. Friends that I'm in contact with on a regular basis have their own folder. I have one called "Clients" and all my clients are listed separately in that folder as subfolders.

(All these folders end up in alphabetical order, by the way.)

I have oodles of folders and subfolders but, hey, I gotta tell ya, that when I need to look something up that somebody sent me or that I sent somebody, I know exactly where I left it.

The more organized we are, even with our computers, the more life becomes fun to live. Live lazy, live large.

Routine or Not Routine? That Is the Question

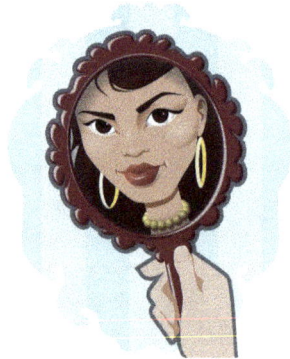

"But if it ain't broke...?"

ROUTINES WILL HELP US REMEMBER WHAT we *need* to remember, like taking our daily medications (that keep us alive), showing up for annual doctors' appointments (which will help keep us alive), eating regular-ish meals (without which we would not be alive for all that long), and so on.

Routines will also give us loads of free time to do whatever we want to do even if, like me, it's only to lie on the couch in the late afternoons and evenings, guiltlessly watching recorded TV shows while napping on and off.

That's part of *my* routine.

This late-afternoon/evening routine of mine doesn't mean I'm lazy. Believe it or not, this doubles as doing writing research. It's "work." I write screenplays as well as short stories and novels, so even watching a movie is "work." A writer's curse? Or a writer's blessing to always have something to do?

My eyes aren't the best anymore, so reading books is difficult. I can't just spread my index finger and thumb apart across a book's pages to increase the size of the type.

So I watch TV programs I can learn things from, or that trigger me to do online searches for obscure scientific, historical or medical stuff. I *can* expand the size of type on my computer screen.

I don't really use my cell phone for anything other than texting, reminders, and being notified of incoming emails. "Business"-related emails I deal with when I'm "at work" in the mornings. I can type a lot faster on a keyboard than I can poke my cell phone's tiny keys with a stick that has little rubber thingey on it. I have my father's spatulate fingertips, plus my years of typing have probably flattened them a tad, too. This makes it difficult for me to operate a cell phone's keyboard. My friends are aware of this so don't expect my usual tome-like replies to their emails in the late afternoons and evenings.

Is there Anything Negative about Routines?

There most certainly is! In my experience, routine can cause madness.

I was once involved with a man who had Obsessive

Compulsive Personality Disorder (OCPD). This is not the same as Obsessive Compulsive Disorder (OCD). https://www.verywellmind.com/ocd-vs-obsessive-compulsive-personality-disorder-2510584

This man I had gotten involved with suffered from "anxiety" (his word), and he controlled my thinking so completely, that within a year, I had a psychotic break. Yes. I did. I sought psychiatric help.

To those of you who know me today, I will say, "No, no, not him. This one goes *way* back."

On the recommendation of my psychiatrist, I suggested to this man that he might want to seek psychiatric help, too. He agreed to attend an appointment with a colleague of my doctor. Therefore, this man was not diagnosed by my psychiatrist *in absentia*, he was diagnosed by an uninvolved professional who knew nothing about me.

My psychiatrist treated me a lot differently after he heard back from his colleague about this man. My psychiatrist set his notebook aside and started teaching me how to recognize OCPD. Thus, I had three years of training with a doctor. Do I know and understand OCPD? I think I do. Do I judge those who have it? I do not. It's a deep-rooted coping mechanism that some people use to survive.

(This man did not pursue psychiatric help beyond the first appointment. And psychiatric appointments were covered by OHIP in those days. This is a symptom of that disorder.)

NOTE: I was raised to be compassionate to all. This can be blinding. Also, if we grow up in a certain environment, we can become immune to noticing warning traits.

The TV program, *Evil Lives Here*, refers to these warning traits as "clues." Missed clues.

ALSO NOTE: I have since been diagnosed as having a "perfectly normal, healthy personality" but was warned, in no uncertain terms, to "stop doing research!" This little old Hungarian shrink (ca. 2005) actually shook her finger at me when she said all this! So now I Google sections of the DSM-5 (https://www.verywellmind.com/the-diagnostic-and-statistical-manual-dsm-2795758) instead of diving in there in person to experience things up close. Bad idea to do that kind of thing first hand! (Yes. I've also gotten myself involved with the odd psychopath, here and there, too. Oh! I could write a book! [*insert laugh track*])

Bottom Line?

If you don't have a routine, start one. If you do have a routine, stop it.

C'mon, Sherrill. That makes no sense whatsoever!

Actually, it does. The idea is to stop doing what we *always* do so we can change things up. Change is always good for us old gals.

Oh. By the way, a routine is not a schedule. A schedule is a straitjacket.

Next post, we'll get started with the first routine: *Don't sleep in.*

"What?" you say, your heart and soul filled with horror at the slightest suggestion of such a thing. "Don't sleep in? Are you out of your mind? Uh. Wait. You said you aren't but... I guess I'll have to wait and see?"

Don't Sleep In

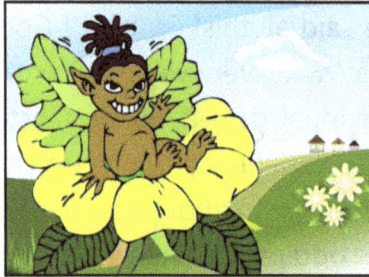

"G' mornin', Sunshine."
(Yeah, right.)

I repeat, Don't sleep in.

Ever.

And stay the hell out of the bedroom except for sleep-time. If we associate our bed with sleeping, that's what we'll do there. (Well, I'm not setting aside what *else* we can do in bed [*winks*], but right now I'm talking about sleeping.)

When we're teenagers, we need a lot of sleep. Sleeping in is important.

But as we get older, we don't need sleep as much. I could never understand how my grandparents could get up at 5:00 every morning. Looking back, I know why my grandfather could. He had to start the furnace or everyone would have frozen to death during autumn, winter, and spring. Grandma had to start the woodstove, no matter what the season, to get the kettle on and start cooking breakfast or everyone would have starved to death.

I don't have a furnace or woodstove to crank up every morning, or a family to feed, but I am up at 6:00. I go to bed around 10:00 PM.

C'mon! Why Not Sleep In?

Sleeping in messes with our circadian rhythm.

What, pray tell, is a circadian rhythm?

"A circadian rhythm (/sərˈkeɪdiən/), or circadian cycle, is a natural, internal process that regulates the sleep–wake cycle and repeats roughly every 24 hours. It can refer to any process that originates within an organism (is endogenous) responds to the environment (entrained by the environment)."

Roughly translated, this means that the circadian of owls and kitty cats for being awake is innately nocturnal (night), and the circadian rhythm of humans for being awake is innately diurnal (day). And this is why kitty cats like to go running around the house in the middle of the night, complaining: "I don't understand why my people feel they have to be sleeping when there's living to be done."

So there's a pattern to our lives then.

It's innate for us to sleep for a certain length of time, and to be awake for a certain length of time. (NOTE: There *are* people who can function on only a few hours' sleep. One of them is a good friend of mine who says her mother and her sister are the same, so it's possibly (probably?)

something in the DNA.)

If we sleep in, let's say, for half an hour, our bodies will still want to stay awake for the usual length of time. That is, if we sleep in for an extra half hour one morning, we'll be wanting to stay awake for an extra half hour that night. It won't be as easy to fall asleep at our regular time (by the clock). And since our bodies are accustomed to sleeping for that certain length of time, we will want to sleep *in* for that extra half-hour (by the clock) the next morning.

Keep sleeping an extra half hour every morning? We will soon be sleeping half the day away and staying up half the night with the cat. (Not that being with the cat is a bad thing, don't get me wrong.)

So What's the Big Deal?

Our sleep habits are not only about sleeping. They also involve when we take our medications—which, by the way, I would think should be taken on a regular basis?

I take thyroid medication. I take it in the morning first thing. I wake up about 6 AM. If I wake up at seven tomorrow, my system will have missed an hour in there. If, tomorrow, I take it at seven, then the next day take it at six, won't I be overlapping?

Think of a gas tank getting completely empty. This will include all the pipes and tubes leading to the motor. We can't just fill up the tank and crank 'er up, we have to mess around until the pipes and tubes get filled with gas, too. Then and only then, will the motor start. Coughing and hacking and complaining as it does. (At least, motors in "my day" worked like that.)

What if we usually fill our gas tank with such-and-such amount of gallons as per our regular habit but it's not quite empty yet. Oops. Gas will overflow all over the pavement at the gas station and if somebody passes by and flicks a match or a cigarette even close to where the fumes are a-rising... Yikes! (This latter take is intended to be an analogy for "overdosing.")

So, smart-ass Sherrill, how do *you* manage to get up at the same time every morning?

I have a Lumie Bodyclock that wakes me up in the morning like dawn would, by gradually brightening from about 5:15 (changeable by the user) until the alarm (annoying little birds), starts chirping at 6:00. The sound is changeable.

Here's a picture of "My Precious":

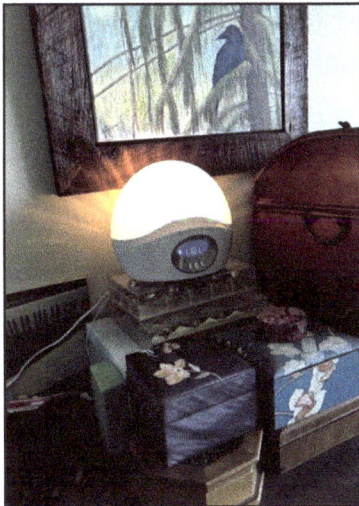

(I just cranked up the light now to take the picture so it shows 11:01 AM. Also, yes, that's a toothbrush behind the Rottweiler figurines on the left. I'll be using it later when I do my regular aquarium maintenance. Then I'll put everything away until next week. Like a good girl. [*insert smiley face*] (I use toothbrushes for things other than brushing my teeth and cleaning aquarium filters. Watch for future posts.))

I almost always wake up before the little birds do and hit the button to ensure they don't start chirping. (They're annoying.) The light stays on.

Incidentally, the Lumie Bodyclock* can be set in the evenings to gradually have the light *dim* over a certain length of time to trigger our melatonin supplies to kick in and help us drift off into sleep. I don't use it. When I go to bed, I go to sleep almost instantly.

I think there are most likely other types of clock that do the same thing. I'm referring to the Lumie Bodyclock because that's the one I use.

The lightbulbs *will* burn out eventually, but are replaceable. I always keep a backup supply of everything I might need. (Future post about that, too.)

In the rest of my apartment—because I have plants and a big-ass aquascaped aquarium in the living room—I have my lights set on timers. This is as much for me as it is for my earth-bound and water-bound plants. There's nothing like heading out of the bedroom to the kitchen in the equivalent of broad daylight at 6:00 AM.

---

*Lumie Bodyclock is available from the actual Lumie site https://www.lumie.com/collections/wake-up-lights as well as other places.

NOTE: When I did the search for "circadian rhythm," up popped links to "circadian rhythm disorder" and "circadian rhythm syndrome."† These are real issues for some folks and these conditions need professional help. But sleeping in and staying up half the night is normally by *choice*, so let's stop messing up our systems like that! It can cause a lot of health issues that we tend to blame on Old Age. Poor Old Age. She gets blamed for darned near everything and it's often our own fault when things start to go awry.

Get an Alexa and ask her to remind you of things "This is a reminder. Yo. Sherrill. It's 7:30. You can't stay in bed all day. Get your ass up and moving."

I will be covering what I hope will be helpful ideas on waking up on time and going to bed = to sleep on time in future posts, as well as how to have a blissful sleep.

_____

†https://www.merckmanuals.com/en-ca/professional/neurologic-disorders/sleep-and-wakefulness-disorders/circadian-rhythm-sleep-disorders#:~:text=Circadian%20rhythm%20sleep%20disorders%20are,Treatment%20depends%20on%20the%20cause.

Getting Started with Routines

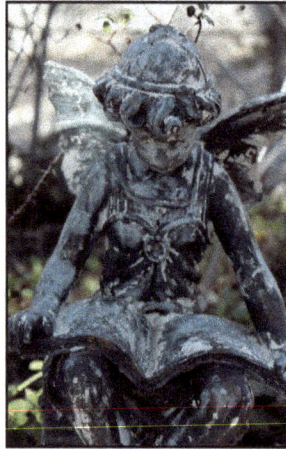

"Locked in stone?"

WHY IS IT, ON MONDAYS, WE wake up saying, "Noooooooooo? It can't be Monday! I'm so tired!" But on Fridays we said, "Yay. It's Friday. I can stay up half the night for the next two." Good way to mess up our timing. We need to stick to the same wake/sleep timing to maintain our mental health. We no longer have to get up to go to work, do we?

Same with our meals. Now I'm not saying we should be eating on a regular basis, like clockwork, like we had to do in the old days when we were 3Cs. Not at all. In fact, I'm what they call a grazer. Much healthier than sitting down three times a day filling our stomachs, and feeling the urge, for the in between times, to reach for a cookie, ice cream or candies. A grazer "reaches for" whatever they have the urge for, no matter the time of day. Freedom!

IMPORTANT: We will need to train ourselves to "reach for" what our body is *needing* and not what we've trained it to think it needs, like sugar and other addictive additives put into ready-made products. Salt is a necessary baddy (iodine source, plus chemically necessary for making bread, for instance); and since it makes food taste good (check out competitive chef shows on TV!), ready-made and take-out tends to have lots of it. The only way to change our food-intake routine is through research, and eating what our body needs for as long as it takes to make us crave the beneficial stuff rather than what will eventually kill us. Read the labels; research each ingredient; watch a year's worth of *How It's Made*.

NOTE: Back in the 1980s when I was seeing the shrink who was teaching me how to recognize OCPD, he recommended that I cut back on salt. I did. My PMS and migraines went away and never came back. To this day, I'm careful about my salt consumption.

Hunger pangs: https://www.healthline.com/health/hunger-pangs#dieting

Regular meals came along when those dudes, those "kings" I mentioned in a previous post, started forcing us to work for them from dawn till dusk. (They must have allowed us breaks to eat or the human race would have disappeared long ago.)

Routines? But I'm a Rebel!

Living by "The Rules" reminds me of growing up in my small home town and having every damned nosy old biddy watch my every move and report it with disdain to my mother. Who then "dealt" with me about it.

Did I have delusions of grandeur thinking everybody in town was watching me? No. I was the eldest of three (and I was an only child until I was nearly six). It was my father's home town, his mother's home town, and the town Dad's great grandmother immigrated to from Ireland with, according to family lore, five children. And Dad was the Chief of Police. Did everybody know me? Everybody knew me. And everybody had opinions of how I should behave.

Funny thing is, I always did "behave" because it's in my nature to be kind, caring and obedient to the Law. Besides, Mom would give me a good smack upside the head (literally) if I didn't behave, and I was a quick learner.

I also—speaking of rules—grew up Roman Catholic. All the way from Grade 1 to Grade 13. But my mother was a convert to Catholicism. Maybe this was why the nuns watched my every move, and corrected my [seemingly] every action? My mother's family were Catholic dislikers. (I don't like the word "hate.") Was this why *they* watched my every move? Did they hope I would self-combust if I walked into a church that wasn't a Catholic one? (Don't laugh. I believed this myself until I was an adolescent; until my cousin got married and I didn't catch fire when I attended her wedding in a Protestant church.) Oh, and Dad's father (a descendant of Northern Ireland Protestants) was a con-vert to Catholicism, too. And Grandma on that side was an

Acadian descendant, not exactly a by-the-church-rules gal, either, although staunchly Catholic. I kept those nuns nosy for sure! Can you figure out where the rebel in me comes from? DNA maybe?

Routines? Rules? Regulations? The mere suggestion of these things today makes me want to run away screaming. But I know that the more organized I am, the faster I can get things done. The faster I can get things done, the more free time—fun—I'm going to have.

Key word: organized. *Not* controlled.

Time to Alter Routines from Bad-for-Us to Good-for-Us

"But I've Never Followed a Routine."

No matter how we deny it, we already follow a routine.

Even running one's life in a chaotic manner is following a *routine* of chaos. It's still a routine.

NOTE: Chaos Addiction is a very real condition arising (usually) from a childhood of constant terror and worry stemming from the need for real or imagined self-protection. It's not an addiction to the terror and worry, but an addiction to the substances produced in our bodies *in response* to the fear and worry. There are those who refer to people with this condition as being "chaos junkies," but this is unkind. Like any addiction, it can be stopped, but not without leaving the feeling of being—according to what I've read—"dead." Where's the motivation, then, to "fix" something like that? In lieu of judging, understand.

I don't plan to get into the deep and dark of various mental disorders like OCPD (Obsessive Compulsive Personality Disorder) and Chaos Addiction, etc. I'm not a psychiatrist. I'm talking about embracing routine in our *lives* so we can *live* a little for a change.

First thing I do when I wake up (around 6:00 AM, give or take by anywhere from ten minutes to half an hour or more, either way) is head for the bathroom. That's often what wakes me up in the first place.

I make my bed.

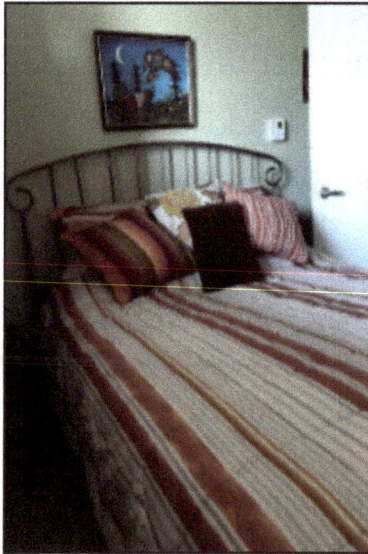

Pull up the duvet. Arrange the pillows/cushions. Bingo. Twenty seconds?

If you have a duvet, all you need to do is pull it up over the sheet that you just pulled up. If you use "hospital corners," it will work much easier as you won't be having everything coming apart at the bottom end. Frustrating and time-consuming.

Anybody can do it: https://www.artofmanliness.com/ articles/how-to-make-a-bed-using-hospital-corners/ #:~:text=Make%20a%20hospital%20corner%20on,fold%2 0the%20top%20drape%20over

I get dressed.

I turn on my cell phone's sound. (My cell phone remains silent from bedtime to dawn. It's plugged in to recharge during this time. It's at my bedside, in case.)

I take my thyroid medication. This has to be taken either one hour before food, or three hours after. I choose the shorter window. I'm a grazer.

I check on the dudes in the small bedroom aquarium: plants, shrimp, and three snails named Waddy, Ithy and Sali (Arabic nicknames for "One" and "Two," and nickname for Salvatore). These are Nerite snails and they like to go exploring, as in, climb out of the aquarium. Stressful for me? Yes. Light comes on at 6:00 AM. It turns off at 1:00 PM. I now dose it with carbon (see more below about this).

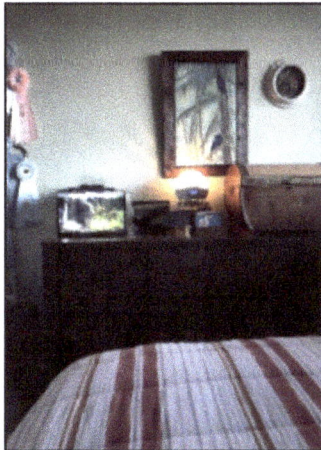

I say good morning to my plants in the rest of the apartment as I check on them: balcony ("Good morning, world!"); or on windowsill in winter. Good morning world again as I open the draperies.

I take my emphysema puffer. Brush my teeth. No point in brushing my teeth, taking the inhaler, then brushing my teeth again, eh?

I turn on the radio to see if World War III started and I missed it. Or are we up to WW IV yet? No? OK. Let's get to work, then. Or play. Or whatever. My time is now my own to do with exactly as I please.

And what I please to do is...

... get onto my computer and check all my emails. I deal with the ones that are quick to deal with, as in, outright delete for marketers; and respond to clients' questions/ replies/etc., usually brief. I respond to friends' emails (chatty tomes, usually) later, when I'm "off work." If it's my day off, I can dally all I want. Days off can vary. Everything I do outside of my routine "depends."

Then I work: writing or editing or designing or whatever. Since I make commitments to clients and to myself, I tend to work Monday to Thursday on writing or clients' projects so I can meet deadlines. Yes. I give myself deadlines. I try to save Fridays and Saturdays to work on my blog so I can be certain to be at least one or two posts ahead—in case something comes up like the end of The Plague and we can all go party, me without the stress of having Something To Do sitting in the back of my mind, ruining my *fun*.

I consider writing to be fun, so spending a few hours

on Friday and Saturday mornings getting ahead on blog posts, is fun. It's playing. I could be knitting, or going fishing, or running, or anything else that people like to do. I like to write.

I also have the "routine" of weekly water changes on my aquariums. This isn't so much "fun" but it's required in order to have the "fun" of seeing how beautiful they can be.

I like to think of "routines" as being Things That Must Be Done Or. I MUST take my meds... or I'll get sick. I MUST open the draperies for my plants... or they'll perish.

After an hour (see thyroid meds above), I can take the rest of my daily meds: calcium, D, B$_{12}$, etc. Taking my daily (doctor-ordered) supplements is on the list of Things That Must Be Done Or.

When I work, I take breaks, maybe wander around the apartment, stretch, dance, look out the window to readjust my eyes, sing...

I finish work after about four hours. Rarely longer because I'm not 30 years old anymore. Although... See, deadlines, above. Anytime I spend a lot of time on a project, it tends to wipe me out. Especially my wrists. (I have a Dragon Naturally Speaking app that I use for straight-out first-draft writing. I'll get to using its advanced features "one of these days.")

Somewhere in here I go on Facebook to respond to Notifications. I have friends on there. Actual friends. People I've known for years. And cousins. Lots of cousins. Both Mom and Dad came from families with nine children. Ergo, I had over 60 first cousins (some have passed). Having done my DNA through ancestry sites, I am finding even more cousins. Third and fourth and fifth from all over the world. And the further back I go in my tree, the more I am realizing that every human on Planet Earth is a cousin! ♥ Ancestry research is something else that's *fun* to do.

Around 1:00 PM the lights come on for my big-ass aquascaped aquarium in the living room...

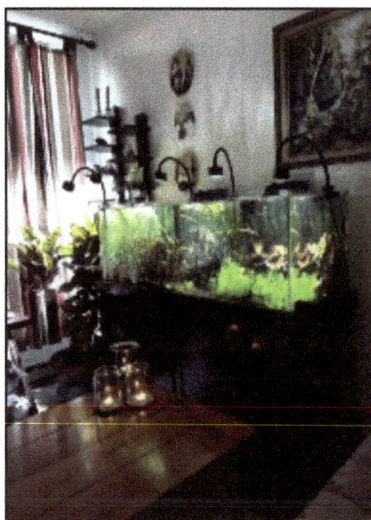

Photo taken early evening, pre Summer Solstice. The really bright lights in the far left corner are for the plant I have named, Queen Croton. (Same lights as I use for the aquarium.)

My other bedroom tank is on until 9:00 PM; the living room tank until just after 10:00 (my bedtime's 10:00). NOTE: I don't think there's such a thing as "only one aquarium." Ask any hobbyist.

The lights for the terrestrial plants are on timers from 6:00 AM to 9:00 PM which is a normal "working day" for them, about 15 hours.

As soon as the aquarium lights come on, I dose with "carbon stuff" (gives the aquatic plants more CO_2, which they require to function when their lights are on). Every Thursday and Sunday, the aquatic plants get fertilizer. There's a medication I take on Thursdays and Sundays, too. I water the terrestrial plants on Thursdays and Sundays. All this "routine" has a twofold benefit:

1. both the plants and I are "dosed" on a regular basis which is healthy; and
2. I have to know what day it is to do this so that makes me remember what day it is.

Normally when we aren't in Plague mode, I go out for a walk. Go for a shop. Run errands. Meet a friend for coffee or lunch. Go on the LRT just for the hell of it. Whatever I want to do. My time is my own and I have oodles of it because I am on a routine for doing Things That Must Be Done Or, so I can get these things out of the way fast.

Woohoo. I'm free.
Free to be me
'cause I'm no longer a 3C!

Nighttime Routines/Sleep Aids, Part 1

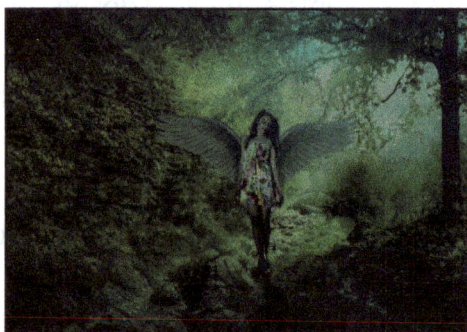

What Day Is it Anyway?

A GREAT WAY OF KNOWING WHAT DAY it is, is by using a medicine tablet thingey. I don't have to keep yelling out, "Hey Alexa, What day is today?" I don't like asking her because she usually adds something like, "Enjoy your day." To this I reply, with my middle finger extended, "Don't tell me what to do."

I refill my medicine tablet thingey on the same day each week. I have to because I will have run out by then.

I have mine set up to be refilled on Mondays, meaning, I have Monday's in there, but tomorrow (Tuesday), I

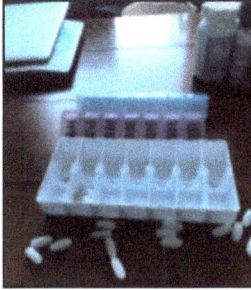

won't have any left. I take my Monday morning meds and then at any time I feel like it during the day, I refill the thingey. Sometimes I refill it on Sunday just because it's nice to get up Monday and it's already been done by the fairies. (Yes, I will have doubles in there on Monday, but I dump the Monday morning bin out and separate the pills, "OK. You two are the same." [slide over with my fingers] "OK. You two are the same." [slide over with my fingers] "OK. You two are the same." [slide over with my fingers]... A little exercise never hurt anyone, right? ha ha)

I take painkillers (hip issues) to get through certain parts of the day, so I set reminders on my cell phone. Eight-hour pain killers at 1:00 PM so any time after 9:00 PM, I can take the ones that will get me through to morning. I pretty much always wait until 10:00 PM for that eight-hour set that will get me through until 6:00. Perhaps this is why I regularly rise at 6:00? My meds have worn off so it hurts to just lie there? I might as well get up, then?

This timing allows for an hour's leeway in case something happens and I miss the 1:00 PM. And no, I don't have to take them exactly on time. Five, ten, fifteen, twenty minutes? Doesn't make any difference *unless they overlap*! Don't overlap painkillers. Ever. (No cell phone to set those handy little reminders with? Get one. Live a little. You're allowed now. You're no longer a 3C.)

I use the 650-dose painkillers and instead of taking two full caplets, I take one and a half. (I have a pill cutter. Any drugstore will carry these.) Sometimes, when my hip is totally killing me and I know I won't be able to sleep well, I take the full two. I sometimes go without during the day, but there's no point in trying to go without at night. I will toss and turn—ow, ow, ow—all night.

Why take more than I need if I don't have to?

It saves money because I won't be using as many.

(It's probably healthier, too.)

Big Hint

I STRONGLY advise against being on a cell phone or computer for at least *two hours* before bed. Sorry.

My apartment is small. My living room is small. My TV is small so it doesn't light up the entire place like an active volcano would. So, if your TV is very large = bright, it might not be a good idea to watch TV for the two hours before bedtime, either.

Why?

Our bodies are constantly doing drugs.

One of the drugs our bodies produce when the lights go out is melatonin. Melatonin makes us sleepy. If we've had our faces in our laptops or cell phones—bright and shiny and gleaming and lovely, "My Precious"—it's going to take a lot longer for the melatonin to kick in.

NOTE: Some people actually take [extra] melatonin to help them sleep. Please, please, please check with your doctor before you try this stuff. As mentioned, I deal with seasonal depression (suicidal depression) so have done a ton of research on "lights" and their effects on Earthlings.

Somebody did an experiment. I'm not certain who did this, and my doctor hadn't heard of the research either, but I am not going to be taking any chances on this. They gave melatonin to people with depression. And it made them suicidal. Oops. Dayum. So be careful with that stuff. With *ANYthing* that isn't prescribed by a legitimate doctor who knows what's s/he's doing, or recommended by a pharmacist. Promise?

More Sleepy-Bye Hints

I turn my covers down around 8:00 PM.

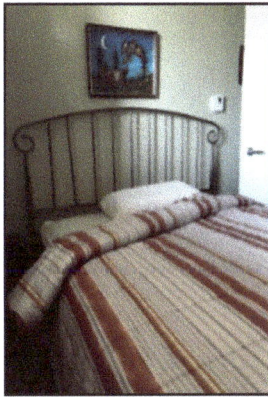

Doing this makes it feel like I have servants or something, like I'm a princess. And every time I walk past my door, it seems to trigger something in me that makes me want to go lie down and sleep. But I have to wait, don't I? Did you notice that psychological trick there? Denial triggers desire.

(For those who suffer from Chaos Addiction, you might pretend that prison guards have been checking for contraband drugs or weapons, or bedbugs. NOTE: I'm being serious. I'm not making fun of anyone. That's not me.)

Another thing I do before bedtime, is make sure there are no dishes in the sink. Big benefit of doing dishes as you go, during the day, is that when you wake up in the morning, there's nothing in the sink except maybe that one water or wine glass—that's sitting there with a wee dollop of dish soap and water in it so has been soaking (cleaning itself) overnight, right? The fairies were here. You don't have to get up and start cleaning something right away. Yay. So why not get out of bed and get the day started?

Nighttime Routines/Sleep Aids, Part 2

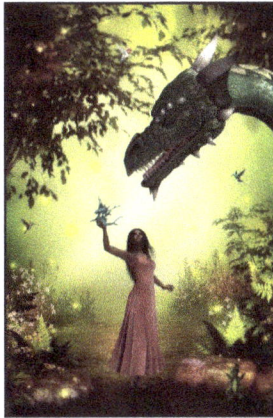

TV or not TV?

IF YOU DECIDE THAT WATCHING TV won't be too en-*light*-ening for you (sorry), make certain you watch something pleasant on TV, not something wild and exciting and action filled that will stay with you, "If only he'd slammed that opponent into the boards, he would have gotten the goal." Make it something that you know will have a satisfying, soothing, calm (boring?) ending so when you go to bed, you'll have a peaceful, easy feeling to start with as you begin to file away.

File away? What's she talking about? "To file away"?

Believe it or not, our brains spend most of the night filing away our day's activities. (Yup. Our bodies are on their own drugs and our brains are Suzie Secretaries.) Once everything has been filed away to the satisfaction of our amygdalae, we can drift away into sweet dreams.

There she goes again. Amygdalae? What the hell is that?

I like to refer to my amygdalae (singular, amygdala) as the little guard dogs in my brain. We've all got them. I wrote about them in my book, *How to Write a Book: Park It, Get to Work,** but here, I'll just provide a link.

https://www.neuroscientificallychallenged.com/blo g/know-your-brain-amygdala

The amygdalae like to make their own decisions based on stuff that scared the sh*t out of them when we were little kids. They remember that stuff for.e.ver! That's why we have dreams. Nightmares! Things get symbolized easily in our heads. Even forgotten. I knew a guy who could shoot the neighbor's dog one day, sleep on it, and wake up the next morning and it never happened. Yep, his amygdalae were that good.

But most of us are kind, loving people without a single psychotic twitch in our minds. And we *can* reprogram our amygdalae. They ain't gonna like it, but it most

---

*https://www.amazon.ca/How-Write-Book-Park-Work/dp/1987491343/ref=sr_1_1?dchild=1&keywords=sh errill+work+how+to+write+a+book&qid=1625229374&s r=8-1

certainly can be done. (Chaos Addicts take note.) This can be done through what is called "breaking our programming." I did it. Anybody can. Like everything else, we just have to *want* to. (The magic wand is "want.")

Now. Where was I? Ah.

What we do when we go to sleep is file the day's activities and after that's done, we can drift into calm, healing sleep. If we have watched something disturbing or overly exciting on TV that is keeping us thinking about it, our Suzie Secretary needs to spend time trying to file that. (She might even give up and just bury it in a hidden spot where it will eventually cause havoc to our health. Anything not filed away properly will fester.)

NOTE: If we miss sleep and don't do our filing, it will continue to pile up and pile up and pile up... But, according to my shrink of old, we can catch up on missed sleep (filing) but it can take days, weeks, even months.

Some of the shows I like to watch before bedtime— and I record everything—are: cooking competition shows and sometimes those shows in which these big whonking tow trucks ("rotators") haul 18-wheelers out of the ditch in BC or on Hwy 401. Another one I like is *American Ninja Warrior*. Believe it or not, *American Ninja Warrior* is rather uplifting. Exciting, but uplifting. There's little to file away for any of these shows: (1) they always have a happy ending, and (2) I'm not personally involved.

I do not listen to the news before bedtime, or anything like that. Because these things are "real" (high stress levels), it takes Suzie longer to file them away. Even if I want to know the next day's weather, I ask Alexa: "Alexa? What's the weather tomorrow?" I rarely go onto Facebook in the evenings for the same reason. Cooking competition shows, tow trucks drivers helping people (and each other), and *American Ninja Warrior*, etc. are my big girl bedtime stories.

A spiritual counselor once told me that if something in my life is bothering me, write it on a piece of paper and set fire to it before going to bed. I don't think that would work because then I'd be worrying all night whether or not I put the fire out. Great concept, though. Perhaps we could write it mentally on a mental piece of paper? Someone else suggested this "piece of paper" could be set on an altar. A "mental" altar.

But I Keep Waking Up

Let's make our minds plan projects during those times we awaken.

When our mind starts wandering off into Worryland (Amygdalae Land?), our sleep (= our health) is greatly affected in a negative way. It ages us before our time.

I've mentioned before that I'm a writer. When I wake up in the middle of the night, I work on the next section of my current work in progress or try to think of what my next book could be about. That always puts me to sleep. Work, eh?

I used to be an avid knitter so I would plan projects in my head. (I liked to design my own patterns.) This might work for the non-writers among us.

Our amygdalae like us to join them when they rehash all those "horrible scary things" we "put them through" during the day. They need to exaggerate so they can keep us in Terror Mode. Keeping us in Terror Mode makes it much easier to control what we do; they like to keep things exactly the same way things have always been. "No changes, please! I will surely DIE if you change anything!" Tell them to go take a hike. Or tell them, "There, there. Everything's under control. We got this." Maybe tell them you're busy re-designing the Suez Canal in your head, or something. And then do that.

Oh. One fun thing I like to do is try to spend a billion dollars. And no, you don't give it away to charity or go on trips with it (right away, at least), you build homeless shelters; you design your new house with its servants' quarters (mine would require that I convince four of my neighbors to let me buy their houses and tear them down to make room for my gigantic new one—I like my neighborhood, I don't want to leave it); you figure out how to set up the schedules for the bodyguards—and how many bodyguards—you're going to be needing 24/7 without having to make any of them work overtime; and they need yearly vacations and sick days and kids-are-sick days; same thing with the chauffeurs you're going to be needing; you add as many two-, three- or four-bedroom apartments required for your now-enormous staff (and NOT minimum-wage staff, either, right?) and their families to live in... (This is already making me nod off and I'm not even in bed!)

Is It Easy?

We can't just "get into the habit" of going to bed and falling asleep right away. We must change entire thought processes. We've programmed ourselves—been programmed?

—to live a certain way. A way we don't have to anymore. (See, breaking our programming above.)

Remember: For us old dolls, there's no such thing as weekends anymore. Or "regular" meals that were geared to school and work schedules. Let's change it up! Let's celebrate. Let's spend as much time in the sun (the schedule of the Sun) as we can! And especially, let's sleep well.

What's Next?

Over the next few posts, I'll cover more routines that will help free us from routine: little tricks I've learned over the years to save time and energy for things other than cooking and cleaning. (Hint: "<u>C</u>ooking" and "<u>C</u>leaning" are two of the Cs in 3Cs.)

However, I have only so many [I hope unique] ideas to share. There's no point in sharing hints that every one of us old ladies was trained to do by the time we were twelve years old. But I'll try.

These routines of mine allow me time to do what I like to do for fun:

I do volunteer work for a dog-rescue group and just received one of their annual, time-sensitive projects a couple of days ago.

I have started writing a new book. (Between Kesk8a books,* I usually write something in another genre.) Work-

---

*Book four in the Kesk8a series is *Hanged for l'Acadie*. Two more books in the series to go then no more self-torture

ing title of this one is "Maureen Tries Online Dating." Maureen is, like me, in her seventies. Like me, she has tackled dating sites. She finally finds one she likes but she accidentally kills him by sneaking a certain "enhancement" into his wine. And now, with the help of her BFF, she has to dispose of the body. But if Maureen thought that was her biggest problem, she's got another think coming.

And I simply MUST get back into ancestry. I set it aside a couple of years ago to get Book #3 of my Kesk8a series done and to get going on #4. (#4 has been published. (Yay!)) I'll be starting Kesk8a #5 maybe end of December (2021). I have to squeeze ancestry in there somewhere! Since The Plague had folks staying in lockdown, I am seeing many, many more lovely little leaves on my tree. (On the ancestry.com site, a leaf = a hint.) I can almost hear my neglected tree singing the popular song from that now *extremely* politically incorrect old movie, *Rose Marie*: How did that go? Oh, to paraphrase: "I am calling you ooh ooh ooh ooh ooh ooh." And "I must answer too ooh ooh ooh ooh ooh ooh."

---

researching things done to the Indigenous peoples and to my ancestors, the Acadians, ca. 1680–1755 back in l'Acadie/ NovaScotia.https://www.amazon.ca/Death-lAcadie-Kesk8a-Sherrill-Wark/dp/1511501154/ref=sr_1_11?dchild=1&key words=sherrill+wark&qid=1625230461&sr=8-11

Hints and Tricks for Gettin' 'er Done, Part 1

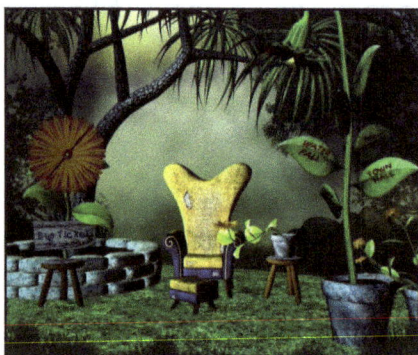

It feels so good when it stops.

I LIKE WATCHING TV IN THE LATE afternoons and evenings. I'm up at 6:00 AM. My "work" is done and over by 2:00 PM at the *latest*. (That's an eight-hour day right there.) I deserve it. I deserve to be able to just—as my mother would call it—"sit around on my ass." (When I was a kid, she would tell me to "get outside and get some of the stink blown off." That still makes me laugh.)

So I record everything. I will be grateful forever to a friend, a son from another mother, for giving me the idea. (♥ Troy! ♥) I don't have to worry about missing any of my favorite shows anymore. Or, to put it another way, saving myself from death by boredom.

My TV provider allows me to record several shows simultaneously in the background, whether my TV is on or off.

Advantages:

- if I nod off—er, *when* I nod off—while watching a program, I can rewind;
- I can save several episodes and binge watch—or not;
- I can go for a walk, go out to lunch/dinner, go visit relatives and friends at any time of day, night or week and not stress about missing an episode;
- I can do whatever I want when I want and it will not be geared around program times for fave TV shows. (Not like the old days, eh?);
- **and most necessary of all**, I can fast forward over the commercials.

Why do I find it so necessary to skip the commercials?

Commercials are manipulations that make us (a) spend/waste money on stuff we don't need, (b) re-clutter our abodes, and/or (c) order in food that's going to probably kill us eventually.

FYI, someone told me years ago—I think it might have been a marketing expert giving a talk at one of the places I worked when I was typesetting/graphic designing —that commercials are aimed at the audience the program lures. That is, the marketing experts are controlling us. At least, trying to. They're trying to turn us into mindless, robotic consumers.

Thus, a commercial is a marketing tactic that attempts to make us keep manipulators wealthy. And if you think about it, it seems like "everybody" these days is crying out: "Tax the wealthy." Um. What if we stopped buying stuff we don't need that they sell? That would work, too. Maybe even better?

Enough of my spiel on commercials. This is all leading up to...

Shopping Tips and Tricks

If you buy in bulk, you'll save on:
- cost of product (less $ packaging $)
- time shopping (= more fun doing what we want)
- vehicle fuel/bus fare
- money spent on fast-food (and eventually on medications for resultant illnesses after years of eating fast food, right?)

Oh, and by the way, my fridge's freezer is spacious but I also have a freezer-freezer.

I drink my coffee half caff and half de-caff and this is for safety reasons. (That's a joke, of course, but I do tend to become rather, shall we say, "impatient" when I drink pure caff. And, as I mentioned in another post, there's no point to drinking de-caff.)

Pre Plague I was able to go to a store and buy two equal sizes of tins of pre-ground coffee, one caff, one de-caff. But online, they are only available from two different brands/sources and they come in different sizes. (I'm not pushing the brands in the photo.) To get an equal mixture, I have to order three + two, and this combo actually works out equally. I mix a large "zip" bag's worth and double bagging that, and squishing the air out, I keep it in the freezer until it runs out then I mix another batch from the tins (that I keep in the freezer once opened, too). Not shown: I keep a few days' worth of coffee in a small container beside the big pot there. A few days of exposure to room temp doesn't destroy the taste (entirely).

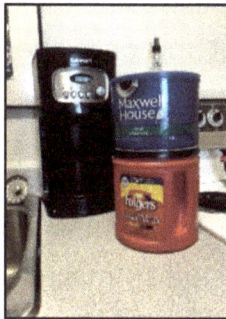

I use filters instead of cleaning the "sieve" thingey in my coffee maker. That's just a personal choice. (Both filter and grounds can go into the compost; filters can be used for many other things according to Facebook posts I've seen; etc.) And I use a big coffee maker not one of those pod ones. A pot can go into the fridge for my iced coffee, or I can reheat mug by mug in the microwave. (If we cover the pot, the coffee tends to stay fresher. I use a dishcloth with a doubled and folded paper towel barrier. Coffee stains.) Of course, I don't have to make a full pot each time.

A general rule is: Don't buy *food* in bulk unless you

are able to either keep it frozen or freeze it yourself. Why not?

If "they" are able to make food (lettuce for example) last for days and days until you use it all up, I recommend you ask yourself what kind of preservatives "they" put into it. Example: Why is it that when I make my own bread it goes stale and starts to grow things very quickly, but when I buy it at the store, it's still lovely and squishy and eatable a week or more later? Hmm. (I slice my homemade bread into... well, slices... but also cut the end portions into "buns," then into the freezer it goes. Note to self: Save up to buy one of those actual bread slicer things. My slicing abilities are slim to none! But the only one around to complain about it is moi.)

I highly recommend getting a bread maker. It's totally cool to make bread, buns, pizza dough, pasta dough... And it's obviously healthier than consuming whatever "they" put into stuff to make it "last longer." (I won mine in a contest years ago for my poem, "Grandma's Bread.")

Remember at the beginning of The COVID Plague, yeast was as hard to find as toilet paper? I still have a lot of yeast left from the two-pound bag I ordered online. (It was the only choice.) I make sure I close the bag tightly after each use—squish the air out of it—keep it wrapped tightly in two plastic lunch bags, then inside a "zip" bag in the freezer. (I should write a horror story some day about yeast, eh? About how you can freeze it and it's still aliiiiiive, two years later...)

Thank you, oh great big huge bulk seller company

that we can order absolutely anything from online and who shall go unnamed! ♥ (In my defense, I have no car and since I have emphysema (if you don't smoke, don't start), I can't wear a mask, so taking public transport is out during The Plague. I'm now double-vaxed but not everyone else is, so...)

Buying in bulk means you'll always have a spare on hand = no pressure to go shopping. As mentioned in a previous post, I take doctor-recommended vitamins, and pain killers. I always have one unopened bottle as a backup. The moment I open the second-last bottle, I purchase a new one.

Same with anything I can't get by running across the street to the corner store.

Use facial tissues for quick swipes instead of paper towels. Pluck versus (1) grab, (2) position, (3) tear = time saved. (Thank for that trick, my dear friend ♥ Pat ♥.)

The paper towels that let you select the size you need, last longer and this means less shopping, less money paid out. Like foil wrap, paper towels *can* be re-used, *depending*. I set aside a paper towel that I might have used only to dry something with. Meaning, it's still clean. Later, I can use it to wipe something off with (like the floor when I drop something), then dispose of it.

I buy my milk in bags from the corner store and freeze them. NOTE: Take great care not to bang the frozen bag on anything. I thaw them in a "plastic box" container, just in case they spring a leak. It has happened to me. Then I put the bag into a milk holder thingey and snip the top corner.

Very often, when these bags come out of the fridge, especially in summer humidity, they won't go all the way into the holder thingey. This is where chopsticks come in handy. Take two chopsticks and stuff one into each side of the holder thingey and slide them back and forth GENTLY alongside the bag of milk. This will release the bag and allow it to slide down.

I keep my supplies in big plastic containers. That way, I know exactly where they are. No excuses.

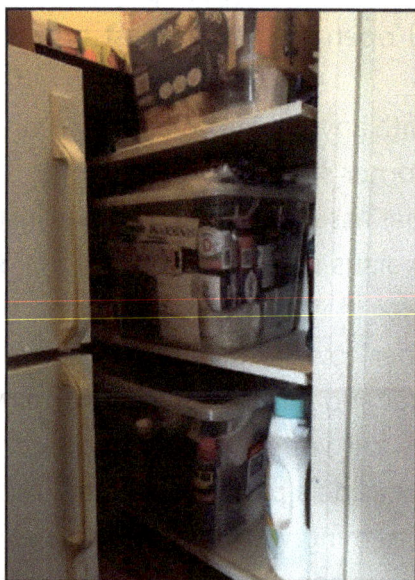

And yes, that's a fridge. When I moved in here, I brought my own with me. The landlord wouldn't take theirs out so I put it in my storage area and use it as a pantry. Hey, why not, eh? I store my flour, sugar, and other things that might draw "unwelcome visitors" into my inner-city apartment.

A Couple of Hints

Cut off the top bit of a frozen vegetable bag and use that as a tie.

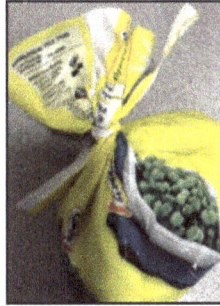

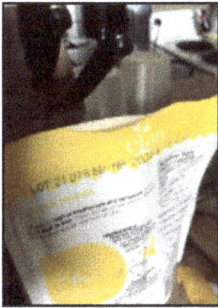

After trimming off the top of a bag like the one below—the ones that zip closed—trim a "curve" on one side so you don't stand there for 10 minutes trying to open it the next time. (See above: Why I don't dare drink pure caff coffee.)

A Shopping Thought

Do I extra-shop because I'm lonely or, bored? Do I shop because I'm a shopaholic? Or do I shop because I'm out of stuff?

Throw all that guilt aside, ladies. And instead, let's program ourselves to resist our very natures. Yes. It can be done.

Remember my previous post when I mentioned hunting and gathering? That the females did pretty much all the gathering because they were "back home at the cave looking after the kids"?

It's in our DNA to gather. The only disadvantage these days is that it's not free for the gathering anymore. We need to learn how to resist the commercials. It can be done. Easiest way, like I said at the beginning of this post, is to record all your TV programs and fast forward over the marketing ploys. (I can hear rumbling in the background from the marketers but to that I reply, "Too bad so sad" and stick my tongue out at them.)

GRANDMA'S BREAD

Old fingers knuckle deep in dough,
Floured kisses age my youthful hair.
Grandma's making bread, you know.
Odours linger in my mind somewhere.

Now my old hands form silk-smooth mounds,
And memories of Grandma's love back then,
Images of crisp, gold, buttered rounds
Rejuvenate, make me young again.

© 1998, Sherrill Wark
Winning poem in a *CJOH Noon News* contest, read by Leanne Kusak, co-host. Prize: a Black & Decker breadmaker.

Hints and Tricks for Gettin' 'er Done, Part 2

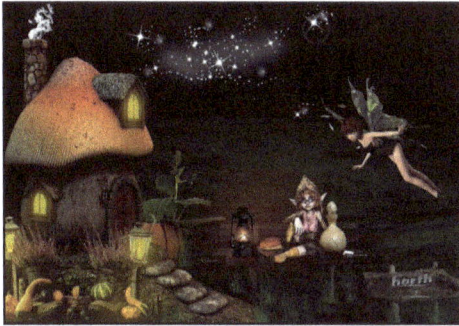

Much better, yes?

WELL, LADIES, THIS IS MY FINAL post. Not my final-forever post, I hope, just my final post for Live Lazy, Live Large: Tips for Making Life Fun for Us Ol' Ladies.

I've written other blogs (mostly about writing and now in book format) as every now and again, a blog idea strikes me and away I go spending weekends sharing what I've learned on my journey and blah-blah-ing away about this and that.

I could carry on and on and on with household tips but there's no point in overlapping what most of you have mastered since your arrival on Planet Earth. I mean, you could give me ten times as many ideas. If I keep going, I will only start re-waxing the same tables you guys probably have been doing since you were kids.

Hints and Tips

These hints will be in random order. This is to keep you awake and alert while you go through them. [*snort*] Or perhaps to be annoying to readers who insist on order. Which I have been saying all along not to do; that we must put aside the idea of having to always do everything the same way.

Just do it.

How to exercise: Stand up straight. Straighten your legs/knees. Shoulders back. Feet pointed out. Breathe. Try it for longer and longer each time.

My computer desk has a shelf under the main desktop. (Elbow level. Ex-typesetter Smart Move!) On this, I keep my keyboard. Beside my keyboard is one of those "frilly duster" things. I not only use it on my keyboard but also on my computer screen, desk, printer(s)... Oh, look! I'm passing by the coffee table to go look out the window—remember taking those breaks for our eyes?—I might as well bring the frilly duster with me and get the coffee table and the window sill and... See what I mean? Tada. Some dusting done and out of the way.

Just do it as you see it. Don't say, "Oh, I'll wait until dusting day." Screw that! Get 'er done!

If you have several things to do—and I cut up used paper into handy-sized bits and write on the backs—make a list. Leave the list at your wrist. Do NOT make long lists. Only the "couple of things" you definitely WILL get at "today."

When you have a to-do list set up, do the sh*ttiest thing first.

Another hint along those lines is, when you have several things to do that are similar, like shelling peas or snapping beans, organize these into "length of time required" and do them from longest time required to shortest. That way gives us hope.

You don't have to like it. You probably won't like it. Just get 'er done.

One new hobby might be to try making different recipes from different cultures. If it turns out that you don't like it, you'll be the only one complaining.

When I say different recipes, I mean from scratch. Example: I make my own hummus. I soak my own chick peas overnight. I cook them myself. I also make my own tahini that goes in it. (Tahini is sesame seed paste.) Toasting sesame seeds is one of the most exciting (read, stressful) things I've ever done in the kitchen. Ditto toasting pine nuts. Chaos addicts take note.

I make my own pasta sauce from canned tomatoes. (NOT the cans that have been pre-flavored (= salted all to hell!) but the plain ones.) I used to grow my own tomatoes when I lived in the country.

Making things from scratch eliminates aaaalllll that toxic crap "they" put into food now to addict us to their brands.

By the way, food does NOT equal love! Food equals

calories. We need only so many calories per day to sustain life. Back in my New Age days, someone told me that when we are babies if, every time we cried, no matter what was going on—a pin stuck in us, actual hunger, boredom, fear, etc.—our mothers just popped a bottle into our mouths, we would forever reach for food (or drink) when anything bothered us. (Think about that one, eh? Yikes!) And this, too, would program us to associate food with "love" even though it wasn't love at all, it was Mom's inexperience (bless her heart).

Back in... I think it was 2008, I was way over my recommended weight. I had stopped smoking and had gained 80 pounds. I'd actually been anorexic since my teen years, a walking skeleton with skin, so it was kind of exciting when breasts sprouted—Wow! What are those things?—but then everything else sprouted too. Eek!

What did I do?

I used my head. I found out how much I should weigh for my height. Then I found out how many calories I needed to maintain that weight. Then I cut that number in half and went all OCPD on reading labels and researching the calories of everything that was going to be entering my mouth...

NOTE: You will freak out totally when you read what actually is in "food." They will list salt. Then they will list "flavoring" which includes salt again. I recommend a TV program called, *How It's Made*. Just Google it. I think you might be able to download episodes. But be prepared to be grossed out when they show how food is made. Dog food is a thousand times healthier and that's because we love them. Should we not love ourselves, too?)

Then I ate whatever the hell I wanted to eat but kept it under the 1,200 calories per day. Example: Instead of hotdogs with buns, I trimmed off the crusts from actual bread and wrapped my dogs in that. Bingo. 100 calories for that "snack". (I mentioned in a previous post that I'm a grazer.) I went only by calories. That was it. Nothing else. I ate what I wanted. I had ice cream daily. But only a wee bit at a time. Six "meals" at 200 calories per = the 1200 calories I was allowing myself. Twelve "meals" at 100 calories per...

Within four months I had lost 40 pounds. I was now at what I should weigh. No more anorexia. I finally had breasts! No more eating to fill a void. I was in total control of me! Yay.

The more you dislike something, the sooner you need to get 'er done and out of the way.

From an episode of the TV series, *Forged in Fire*: "With that many years of experience, you learn to work smarter instead of harder."

Most of the hints and tricks here are well-nigh impossible unless we live alone, but do not ever play the blame game. The blame game makes humans bitter and maintaining bitterness inside can cause illnesses. (Scary, yeah. But true.)

Wipe out the microwave after every use. My microwave's door opens down. Look at all that moisture on the door! (Next page.)

I keep a clean/separate dishcloth at hand and use it pretty much every time. (One thousand and one, one thousand and two.) Hey. My microwave is state-of-the-art

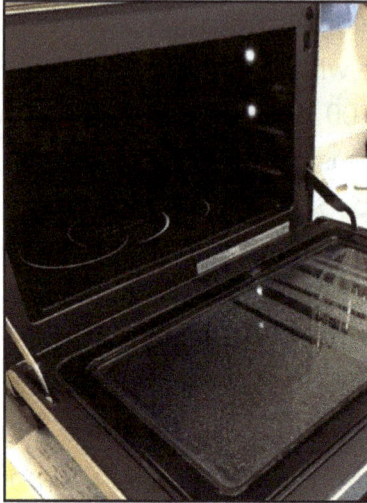

= $$$ so I want it to last as long as possible, right? Remember the term "built-in obsolescence"? I wipe the sides, too, if there's a lot of extra moisture. (One thousand and three, one thousand and four, then one thousand and five for the "ceiling.")

By the way again, I can't use my apartment stove's oven. No matter how I clean it, it sets off the fire alarm. (Long boring story about why I won't ask for a new one. It's OK. It's OK. I'm good.) Ergo, I use my microwave which is also a convection oven, a steamer and a griller. Hey. Why not, eh? But it's tricky to do cakes in. But since I rarely bake cakes anyway...

Speaking of moisture and how moisture can cause damage, we might as well clean the shower stall walls while we're in there, right? I keep a sponge—yes, one of those "enchanted sponges"—and wipe the walls as far up as I can reach every few showers or so. (But be sure to hold onto the bliddy railings when you're doing this! If you don't have railings in your shower "at your age," get some installed! Very important. When we old ladies break a hip, it's downhill into the grave from there. Seriously!)

Take a minute to save two.

Don't make a mess in the first place. VITAL!

Get a vacuuming robot (mine's name is Cecil) and/or floor washer robot (mine's name is Brendan). But unless we declutter before getting one of these, they'll be essentially useless so a waste of money.

Laundry ideas: I have lots of undies and t-shirts so I'm not forced to do laundry constantly.

I take the laundry out of dryer right away so it won't wrinkle. If it's still slightly damp—*slightly* damp, never wet—I can spread things out on my bed or couch to dry out better. I prefer to use my bed so I will definitely have to fold them and put them away before I can go to sleep at night. [*winks at mean trick done to self*]

Chop up your dental floss before discarding it. If it goes into the dump as a long string, it can harm wildlife.

Leave "signals" for yourself. Example: Whenever I take my morning meds from my pill thingey, I make sure to have the other side facing out so when I look at it, I will know I haven't taken my evening meds yet. When I take my painkillers, I turn the bottle upside down so I'll know, Yes. I took them already.

This is my breadmaker's pan. (Next page.) It's very hot when the bread is done so I set it aside and put hot water into it to soak the flipper at the bottom of it. The flipper usually has bread stuck on it.

So I won't forget that it needs to be cleaned, I leave the handle pointed away when it's dirty and toward me when it's clean. When I pour in the flour, I always make sure the handle is toward me as I can pour the flour in better that way. Handle close to me? Ready to go.

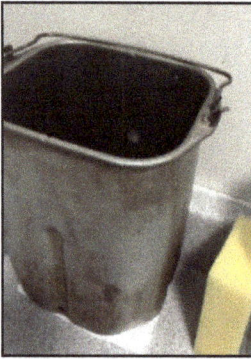

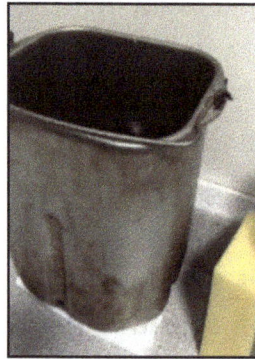

Do things in batches: shop, cook, clean up; a big freezer is important; deep clean spring and fall in one shot rather than haul everything out several times.

Organize Ziploc and Tupperware containers inside bigger ones.

Keep cookbooks in the same place.

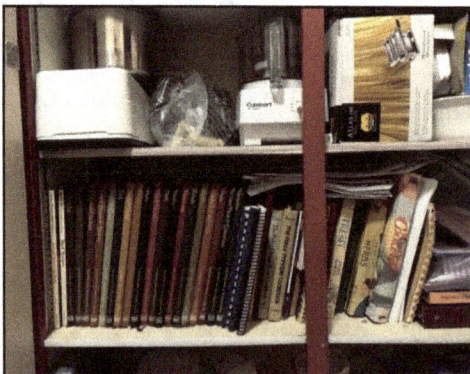

I don't throw out my old electric toothbrushes when they're past their best-by dates but still have power left. I use them to clean around my taps and the edges of my sink(s) and other things. The ones without batteries, I use to clean the filters for my aquariums. Toothbrushes are handy for lots of things. Just don't mix them up.

Clean something when you SEE IT! Not "every Tuesday" after a week's accumulation. 1 min x 7 as opposed to 15 min x 1 is a savings of 8 minutes a week.

Don't leave dishes in the sink. Immediately after use, fill what you've just used with hot water, squirt in a drop of soap, maybe place the utensils inside. Let this soak until you come into the kitchen the next time. Rinse. Dry. Put away. And especially, always before bed! (So it will feel like the elves were in overnight. ♥)

Twice a year, my plants inspire housecleaning. The housecleaning part isn't part of the passion though. Trust me on that. Moving the plants outside toward the end of May leaves that area of my living room clear for moving furniture so I can get in there and deep clean and deep vacuum everything, and wash the big picture window. Before the plants come back in around mid-October, that spot gets another deep clean.

And while I have all that stuff out: vacuum cleaner, water pail, paper towels, window cleaner, floor cleaner, furniture polish, floor wax, etc., I might as well do the whole living room, right? In fact, if I take, let's say, the entire day, I can probably get my entire apartment spiffy-clean to the point where my dear late mother would approve. I'm going to be moving furniture anyway, right? Might as well just get 'er done. (I'm talking about a deep get 'er done when doing this, eh?)

Stop work at "quitting time." Set time limits for yourself and when the clock comes around, "punch out." You don't have obligations to anyone other than to yourself. If you have nothing else to do, start a hobby. (I started aquascaping about three years ago. Four years? I've lost track because of Plague Lockdown. But why not?)

Speaking of hobbies...

Grow plants. I actually have a date tree that I grew from a date pit. Yes I do.

I've tried to grow oranges and tomatoes and other things from seeds, too. Most were not successful because "they" do things to the plants so only "they" can grow them. $$$ But why not give it a shot anyway. It's fun and when they actually sprout, it's such a nice feeling. ♥

Set up an aquarium or aquascape and grow more plants in there.

Start tai chi.

Dance.

Take regular walks. Walk faster and faster and faster until you're able to do that weird Olympic wiggle walk.

Be sure to have your hearing aids in every time you go outside so you can snicker away when people talk about you behind your back,

"I swear that old lady must be right out of her mind. Aren't they supposed to be at home rocking in their chair and knitting or crocheting blankets for their grandchildren or something?"

Salute them with the one-finger peace sign and carry on! ♥

Oh. And as "promised"... What is a 3C? Now remember, this was in my day, and it wasn't all husbands toward all wives, but 3C means, a Cooking, Cleaning, C*m-Bucket.

Fare well, ladies. Live long and prosper.